Living Through Leukemia

Also by Louis George Whitehead

*An Era of Free Native American Press: Tim Giago and the Lakota Times,
Indian Country Today,* and the *Lakota Journal 1981–2003*
Ethel Austin Martin: One Brave Lady

Living Through Leukemia

◆

A Journey to Health

Louis George Whitehead

iUniverse, Inc.
New York Lincoln Shanghai

Living Through Leukemia
A Journey to Health

Copyright © 2007 by Louis George Whitehead

iUniverse books may be ordered through booksellers or by contacting:

iUniverse
2021 Pine Lake Road, Suite 100
Lincoln, NE 68512
www.iuniverse.com
1-800-Authors (1-800-288-4677)

ISBN: 978-0-595-44522-6 (pbk)
ISBN: 978-0-595-68902-6 (cloth)
ISBN: 978-0-595-88850-4 (ebk)

Printed in the United States of America

For Mom

Contents

Acknowledgments

One would think that the experiences of living through leukemia and writing this book couldn't be more different; I see some similarities. One is that I could neither have survived my illness nor written this book without the support and encouragement of so many others. And for that support I'd like to offer my thanks to the following:

The Creator for the strength and understanding to overcome obstacles I have faced during my journey through life.

My mom and dad for their love and for standing by me in all that I have accomplished.

My many friends and relatives who offered their support, prayers, and encouragement during my illness and the writing of this book.

Drs. Robert Nelimark, Philip McGlave, and Kelly McCaul and the many other doctors and nurses who have cared for and treated me since my diagnosis.

Valerian for his prayers and spiritual guidance as I went through the leukemia and the bone marrow transplant.

Steve and Leet for counseling me during some very dark times after the bone marrow transplant.

Marianne and Mary for sharing their content and style suggestions during the writing of this book.

Lee IV, Jay, Richard, and others in the Wordcraft Circle of Native Writers and Storytellers family for their encouragement in putting this book together.

David for pushing me to keep writing and to become a better writer.

Dolly for being my muse and for always believing in me as both a writer and a human being.

Preface

Life before 1999 had always been rather ordinary. It was a good life, but nothing I'd call extraordinary. I was born in an east-central South Dakota town of about eighteen thousand people. The population of the entire state hovers around 750,000.

I was born to a middle-class mother and father who supported themselves through honest labor and did their best to raise their only child. Mom was a Columbus, Ohio, native who worked as a purchasing agent and materials manager at a regional electric cooperative. Dad was a retired electrical engineer. He was born in northwestern Iowa and had worked for aircraft manufacturers around the country before settling and farming in South Dakota after marrying my mother in 1964. Our family was like that of many of my peers except for a few details. Most of the people with whom I grew up and went to school were born to parents in their late twenties or early thirties. When I was born, my dad was fifty-six, and my mom was thirty-nine. Dad is eighty-six now, and Mom would have been sixty-eight if she were still alive. I'm twenty-nine as of this writing.

My birth at that late stage in their lives didn't occur by design; it just happened that way. And while my peers spent most of their high school and college years with other young people, I grew from child to man among older adults. In growing up in such an environment, I always felt as though I walked in two worlds—the world of fun and games that I shared with my peers and the world of grown-up responsibilities and concerns that I shared with my parents and others.

Similarly, I feel that my life is divided into two parts. The first part encompasses all of my life experiences before my leukemia diagnosis and bone marrow transplant. The second part is the life I've lived since the diagnosis. Being forced to face my mortality rocked my world in such a way that my life was cleaved in two. It's as though one life ended and another began that blistering August day in Columbus, Ohio.

More than seven years have passed since I was diagnosed with acute myeloid leukemia. Those years have given me plenty of time to reflect on my experiences in going through leukemia. I won't lie and say that I've fully processed everything that happened during that two-year odyssey, but I can offer recollections of all that happened. This book is the product of those experiences, and I hope that whoever reads it finds enjoyment and inspiration. I can think of no higher calling for this work than it being a tool to help others, regardless of whether they are about to go through what I've gone through, have already gone through what I did, or have loved ones who are going head-to-head with leukemia.

As you read this book, and for the rest of your days, I wish you and those close to you good health, peace, happiness, and love.

1

A Life Change before Leukemia

The year 1999 was a big one for me even before I learned in August that I had leukemia. For the first two years of college, I had pursued a pre-pharmacy major at South Dakota State University. Pre-pharmacy had appealed to me because it would lead to a career in the medical field, and such a career likely would prove lucrative and secure. It was also difficult to pursue, and the challenge appealed to me. As time went on, however, I discovered that I was able to perform well in chemistry, biology, and related classes, but I wasn't enjoying them very much.

Deep down, I wanted to be an English major because I enjoyed writing and had always enjoyed my English classes in high school. There were several times throughout the first two years of college that I had wanted to abandon pre-pharmacy and take up something I loved. Something inside me, however, kept urging me on, saying, "It's OK; things will get better."

By the time I entered the professional pharmacy program at the beginning of my junior year, I realized that being in a career in which I could make a lot of money wasn't enough. I understood that having a career I enjoyed was more valuable. So I left the professional pharmacy program in the fall of 1998 after completing only three days of classes. Choosing to leave the program was one of the hardest decisions I've ever made, but I knew in my heart that I was doing what was right for me.

I enrolled in courses I had wanted to take for fun and to work toward my American Indian studies minor. I also spent time exploring my interests and talking to professors in the hopes of finding an alternative major.

If an American Indian studies major had been available at SDSU, I likely would have majored in it. American Indian cultures and issues were always of strong interest to me. I'm a descendant of many nations, most of which are western European. But I can also count indigenous North American peoples, such as the Anishnaabe, Miami, and Six Nations, among my ancestors. Studying American Indian history and culture, albeit in the academic world rather than the "real world," would be a way for me to learn about the history and cultures of peoples to whom I have ties on both sides of my family but about whom I know relatively little. My formal education on American Indians ended when I completed my American Indian studies minor. But my learning about Native America has continued outside university walls through travel and the forging of friendships with indigenous people around the United States and Canada. And my personal connection to Native America has grown in the process.

The first major I considered was English, but it didn't appeal to me in the way it once had. I then looked at majors relating to computers, but nothing lit a fire inside me.

One afternoon, I went to visit my friend and mentor, Valerian, whom I had met not long before. I had met him through various encounters on campus and through the Native American Club, and in a short time, we began to develop a friendship. Through that growing friendship, I opened up about things that were going on in my life, particularly those pertaining to school. I told him how I had left the pharmacy program, and how I was looking at other majors. When he learned that I enjoyed writing but wasn't particularly interested in majoring in English, he suggested I give mass communications a try.

I went to the journalism department and met with the professor, who, five years later, would serve as my adviser while I worked on my master's degree. We discussed my interests and the careers to which a journalism degree could lead. He suggested some classes I could take in the spring. What he proposed sounded good to me, so I took the plunge the following semester. I enrolled in some basic journalism courses, found that I enjoyed them, and haven't looked back since. Little did I know at the time that my career as a journalism student—and my life in general—would experience "a little interruption."

2

First Signs of Trouble

Anyone who's lived in South Dakota knows that the state experiences a lot of extremes, particularly with regard to climate. It can be bone-chilling cold during the winter months and scorching in the summer. The summer of 1999 seemed searing, especially for those of us in classrooms with no air-conditioning.

I was taking a class called State and Local Government, which was required for SDSU's undergraduate journalism program. It taught us about state and local government, but since we were in South Dakota, where around 8 percent of the residents are American Indian, the course also touched upon tribal government structure.

One July day, the dozen or so of us in the class returned to our seats after doing calisthenics for a minute or two. I'm not sure why, but the professor always made us do some physical exercises at the beginning of each class. I don't know if the exercises made us more alert, but they were kind of fun and helped keep the class casual.

The lecture and ensuing discussions continued as they had on preceding days. Our professor explained some facet of government, and then we talked about it or wrote about it in our journals. I hadn't felt bad that day or previously, but I experienced severe chest pains as I leaned back in my desk.

Am I having a heart attack? I wondered to myself.

Since I was only twenty-one years old and was generally healthy, I dismissed that possibility. At around 230 pounds, I was overweight but didn't figure that my weight could cause health issues at that age. The next thing that came to mind was heartburn. Something I ate must have triggered it. But I hadn't eaten or drunk anything out of the ordinary, and heartburn had never been a problem. In any case, I didn't do the right thing. Instead of going to the doctor and getting checked, I endured the stabbing pains in my chest; they went away after a few days. I don't know what caused the pain, but I now suspect that those pains were among the first symptoms that something was very wrong with me.

It wasn't until early the next month that any unusual feelings resurfaced. During the spring semester, I had been selected by our campus chapter of the Golden Key International Honor Society as a delegate to its international convention in Orlando. The trip would last four days during the first week of August.

3

Body Pain Rears Its Head

I got a late start that morning and barely made it to the airport in Sioux Falls in time to catch my flight to Orlando. Once I received my e-ticket and headed up to the boarding area, I was able to settle down and bask in the fact that I was on my way. I had made it.

The flight plan included a leg from Sioux Falls to St. Louis and one from St. Louis to Orlando. The flight to St. Louis passed without incident, but I'll never forget the flight from St. Louis to Orlando. It was one of the rockiest flights I've ever experienced, possibly from flying over the Gulf of Mexico or from unusual weather patterns. There were several times when I wondered whether we'd make it. I tried to focus on the text of *Demolition Man*, a biography of Sting, but my nervousness made it difficult. My uneasiness was unusual, considering I had been on countless other flights. In fact, I took my first flight when I was about two hours old. I had to be flown to the University of Minnesota medical center for emergency surgery for a collapsed lung. This flight, however, was unusually turbulent. About the only thing that kept me calm was a snippet of a music video that kept playing on the small overhead LCD screens in the DC-10's cabin. The song was a live version of Sarah McLachlan's "I Will Remember You." We touched down within a few hours, and I caught a shuttle bus to the hotel where the Golden Key convention was to be held.

When I arrived at the hotel lobby, there was a long line at the check-in counter. It moved quickly, however, and time passed rapidly when I struck up conversations with other convention-goers. Everyone seemed friendly, and I enjoyed meeting other Golden Key members.

Once I made it through the line and was given my room key, I dropped off my bags, freshened up a bit from the day's travels, and went to a banquet that evening. The room was full. The convention theme related to magic, and I remember the youthful energy of the room and the speakers blaring the Steve Miller Band's "Abracadabra."

The evening's program soon began, and we all took our seats. I felt good in spite of the harrowing experiences on the plane earlier that day, and I enjoyed the conversations with my tablemates. There were probably eight of us seated at each table. Later that night, I returned to my room looking forward to the upcoming three days.

The next morning, I still felt tired in spite of a good night's rest. That wasn't altogether unusual, but the tiredness was more pronounced than usual. In any case, I didn't let it bother me. I went to the sessions in which I had enrolled. They were mostly workshops on professional development.

The fatigue that I noticed when I awoke remained with me for the rest of the day. The tiredness wasn't particularly bothersome, but new sensations arose as the day progressed. Those same sensations over the next two and a half days forced me to spend all of my free time resting in my hotel room.

On the afternoon of the second day, my shoulders, lower back, and hips started throbbing. The pain wasn't overwhelming, but it was certainly uncomfortable. I spent part of that day walking up and down the streets of Orlando near my hotel in hopes that I would feel better. Unfortunately, the walks only made me feel worse. So for the remaining days of the conference, I quietly endured the pain. But I didn't suspect that there was anything seriously wrong. I thought perhaps the high humidity or a viral or bacterial infection was bothering me. I had been in contact with a lot of people from many places, so catching a bug seemed logical.

When the conference concluded and I bade farewell to my new friends, I flew back to South Dakota. The return flight followed essentially the same route as the flight to Orlando but didn't seem quite as rocky. Between St. Louis and Sioux Falls, I finished reading *Demolition Man*. I was also relieved that the pain I had experienced in Florida subsided within a day or so of returning to South Dakota.

4

Reprieve

The day after I returned from Florida, I headed to my post at SDSU's Instructional Technologies Center around eight in the morning. I had been putting in more hours there for the past few weeks because my friend and supervisor, Jim, was on a monthlong vacation. While I was away, all of the servers on SDSU's campus were shut down, including the few we had at ITC.

I walked into the Faculty Multimedia Lab where I worked, and ITC's director approached me hurriedly.

"Louis, what's the password for the server?" he asked excitedly.

"I don't know. Jim doesn't tell me those things."

The director left the FacLab, only to return a few minutes later.

"Louis, what is the password for the server?" he asked again, with desperation coloring his voice. "Where does Jim keep it?"

"I don't know. Jim doesn't tell me these things," I repeated.

I could tell the director's anxiety was peaking. If we weren't able to get our servers back online along with the rest of those scattered around campus, our technology infrastructure would essentially collapse.

He looked at me and said, "I can't believe how one student can shut down an entire university, and I can't believe we let it happen." I didn't know if he was talking about me or someone else.

The director hurried off in search of the password and left me standing there speechless. My heart sank as I digested what he had said. At the same time, I tried to convince myself that short of helping him and

11

others find the password, I had done all that I could have in that situation. Within fifteen minutes, the director located the password, and everything came back online. The friendly atmosphere that usually enveloped ITC soon returned.

Once the server crisis had passed, I returned to my post in the FacLab. Jim was supposed to be back in the office about a week later. The remainder of the day turned out to be fairly quiet. There were a few faculty members who needed my help, but otherwise I spent my time working on software applications in the lab.

After lunch, I started capturing and editing video on one of the lab's PCs. I brought in a drumming instructional video by either Dave Weckl or Steve Smith, captured footage from it into the computer, and edited it for use on the Web. I looked at the clock and saw that it was near quitting time, so I started shutting everything down. That evening I planned to pack for a trip to Ohio that would begin the next morning.

5

"You May Have Leukemia"

The mid-August trip to Ohio would be the second for my mother that year. She had flown to Columbus about a month earlier to attend the funeral of her brother, Pat. This trip to Columbus was for Mom to attend some training for her job as a purchasing agent and materials manager for Sioux Valley–Southwestern Electric, now known as Sioux Valley Energy. The training would take place in one of the meeting rooms of the Fairfield Inn in which Mom and I would stay. My going on the trip had nothing to do with Mom's training; I was going along to take some time off before classes started again and to reconnect with relatives in the Buckeye State.

We arrived in the city and headed for the car rental place, where we picked up a Pontiac Grand Am sedan. Then we went to the home of my cousins Scott and Terri Thompson and their daughters, Megan and Amy. The Thompsons were the Ohio relatives with whom we'd stayed in closest contact. We had a good time visiting the family before we headed to our hotel.

Everything seemed to go well during our first two days in Ohio. Mom enjoyed the training, and I had a good time cruising around the city on my own and with Scott and Terri and the rest of the family. I spent most of my free time traveling to car dealerships and music stores. One of my favorites in the area was (and is) Columbus Pro Percussion. I haven't been in that many drum shops, but Columbus Pro Percussion is impressive.

On the afternoon of the third day, Scott had part of the day off, so he and I ran around a bit. We visited a drum shop near his house. As we walked toward the front door, I noticed a black Tama gong bass drum in the display window. I also noticed a squeezing sensation around the circumference of my chest. It wasn't really pain at that point, but it was an uncomfortable tightness. Still, I felt well enough to play some blue Fibes drums in a practice room while I was there. Even with the invisible vice grip that had a fast hold on my torso, it was fun to sit down behind a drum kit. Scott couldn't hear me much as he stood outside the door to the room in which I was playing, but he was able to watch me through the door's window.

Scott headed back to his place after a while, and I was left on my own. Again, it would have been smart to go see a doctor to get the squeezing in my chest checked out, but I didn't. I resigned myself to cruising around more and then resting in the hotel room. I vividly remember sitting in a traffic jam on High Street. The day was overcast, hot, and sticky. Neither I nor the cars around me were moving. There are few things in this world I hate more than being stuck in traffic jams. Yet, I was content to sit and listen to my new live Kansas tape, and it made the time pass more quickly. Over and over, I listened to the classic track, "Carry On Wayward Son."

Around five, Mom finished her classes for that day. We invited Scott, Terri, and the kids over to the room for pizza. I was relieved that the tightness in my chest had subsided. At the same time, a new pain in my upper right leg had begun to develop. I didn't think too much of it at the time, but I would learn less than forty-eight hours later that it was a sign of serious times to come.

I managed to enjoy myself in spite of the pain. We ordered pizza and hung out in and around the hotel's pool. Scott and I spent most of our time wading, and he shared stories about his time in the navy and living in Hawaii. It was fun to spend time with him and with the rest of our relatives, but the pain in my leg was growing worse. By the time everyone else went home and Mom and I retired to our rooms for the evening, I convinced myself that everything would be all right in the morning.

Boy, was I wrong …

I opened my eyes the next morning and glanced at the digital clock on the stand next to my bed—5:45 AM. After staring at the clock for a minute, I sat up in bed and discovered that the sheets were soaked with sweat. And so was I.

My leg was not better; it felt much worse. My right leg was throbbing with pain like I'd never experienced before. As I sat on the edge of my bed wincing in pain, I felt the need to retch. Since I really couldn't walk, I crawled to the toilet and threw up. I had no idea how bad of shape I was in.

Mom had awakened and came to my bedside to attend to me. There wasn't much she could do other than give me water. I took the water, but I had difficulty keeping it down. Within an hour, Mom called Terri, and the two of them took me to an urgent care clinic near our hotel.

When we arrived, the technicians drew some blood, and we waited for the results. They were inconclusive, but one of the nurses said my heart enzymes indicated that something was wrong with my heart. Not wanting to take any chances, they put me in an ambulance and took me to Grant/Riverside Hospital. The clinic staff hadn't given me any pain medication, so all I could do to take the edge off was grit my teeth and wipe the sweat from my brow.

"Whatever you do, don't drop me," I told the paramedics as they carried me from the ambulance into the hospital. It was the first ambulance ride I had taken in more than twenty years.

Nurses in the emergency room drew more blood and gave me some medication to kill the excruciating pain in my leg.

"On a scale of one to ten, how severe is the pain?" one nurse asked.

Since the pain was unbearable, I replied, "Nine." Not long after our exchange, the nurse reappeared with a syringe full of pain medication. She asked me to turn over onto my left side, and she gave me the injection. The shot itself was painful, but the experience I had following the shot wasn't unpleasant. She had given me a dose of Demerol. I'm not sure that the medication reduced the intensity of the pain, but it made me not care about it.

"Oh, wow … I'm flying," I said drowsily, as the nurse wheeled me into an open room. She explained that a doctor would be in to see me shortly. She also said that the blood test results were inconclusive. The nurse said, however, that there seemed to be an unusually high number of immature white blood cells in my system.

Less than an hour later, the same nurse returned and said that the doctor wanted to keep me at least overnight for observation. I consented. Mom and Terri visited me in my room for a while, and then they left for the remainder of the afternoon. The first night in the hospital, I had a roommate, an older gentleman. The second night, the room was mine alone.

Since my leg still caused so much pain, I was unable to sleep on my side, as I was accustomed to doing. Sleeping flat on my back had never been comfortable for me, but I was able to do so in the hospital.

The following afternoon, a doctor I hadn't seen before came to my room. He wasted few words. The doctor, a man in his early fifties, pulled up a chair and prepared to tell me what was surely something important. His statement was just an educated guess, but it would change my life forever.

"Well, Mr. Whitehead, your blood tests show that your immune system is starting to fail ...," he said, pausing long enough to give me time to think. I could feel my stomach turn and beads of sweat start to seep up to the surface of my skin.

Although I had no reason to think that I would have such a disease, my first thought was, *Is he talking about AIDS?* After all, wasn't a failing immune system usually a symptom of AIDS or HIV, the virus that causes AIDS? Having AIDS, though, made little sense even amidst the anxiety that was welling within me. I had never been an intravenous drug user; I hadn't had any blood transfusions; and I hadn't been sexually active at that point in my life. *No, it couldn't be AIDS*, I decided. But if not AIDS, then what?

"We can't confirm it unless we do a bone marrow biopsy," the doctor continued, glancing down at my hands as I sat upright in my bed, "but there's a good chance that you may have leukemia."

Leukemia ... the thought had never crossed my mind. I knew that leukemia was cancer of the blood, but I had never made the connection between leukemia and immune function. On a larger scale, I had also never considered the prospect of having cancer, especially at such a young age. After all, wasn't cancer something that older people developed? How could a twenty-one-year-old man have cancer?

As thousands of thoughts spun around inside my head, the doctor spoke again.

"Now, since your immune system is going downhill fast, that means we only have about forty-eight hours to move you, if you want to be moved. It's up to you. Do you want to be treated here in Columbus, or would you rather be someplace closer to home?" he asked.

I went with my first instinct: although I would be surrounded by plenty of family in Columbus, I wanted to be closer to home. As I would soon find out, "closer to home" meant Sioux Falls. I told the doctor I wanted to be back in South Dakota, and he set the wheels in motion. The doctor bid me good day, patted me on the shoulder, and left the room. I was alone once again.

There's no question that I was surprised at the news, but I was even more surprised that I didn't take it harder than I had. Everyone reacts differently to learning that he or she may have a disease like cancer. Many, when faced with the possibility that they have just been handed a death sentence, go into shock or break down and start crying. I would have expected that of myself if I were a third-party observer to the scene that had just transpired. But I did not react like that.

Instead of fear or shock, I felt a calm mixed with a sense of dread at the prospect of having to undergo chemotherapy. I had never known anyone who had undergone chemotherapy, but I was aware of the treatment regimen's reputation for making those receiving it lose their hair and become very sick. The thought of dying never crossed my mind. I don't think my lack of concern about death was born of denial; I believe I sensed deep within myself that I would survive. And in drawing from my own spirituality, I felt as though someone or something was protecting me. Regardless of how dark my path became, I was confident that I would be all right. And I knew that action was called for if I was going to beat the disease and not leave my loved ones behind.

Calling my mom and Terri and letting them know what was going on was the next thought that came to mind. Mom and I had checked out of our hotel the morning before, so Mom was staying with Terri. I phoned the two of them at the Thompson house and told them what was happening. I also told Mom that I wanted to call Dad and let him know what was happening. Mom thought that it would be better to hold off on calling Dad until travel arrangements had been finalized. I didn't agree with Mom, but I didn't feel like I was in a position to argue. In the meantime, I called some friends to let them know what was happening. Everyone expressed concern, wished me well, and offered support. And everyone—even Mom—at least appeared calm.

By the next morning, travel arrangements were made. My flight would leave in the afternoon, and I would arrive in Sioux Falls around eleven that evening. Shortly after lunch, Mom and Terri came to my room and helped me get dressed and ready for the journey back to South Dakota. They pushed me in my wheelchair down to the hospital lobby and eased me into the front seat of my cousin Kim Beverly's Ford Windstar minivan. I was still wracked with leg pain, but I took some comfort in knowing that I was on my way home. We arrived at the airport about twenty minutes later; our plane took off within two hours.

It turned out that the flight had two legs: the first from Columbus to Minneapolis; the second from Minneapolis to Sioux Falls. Both flights were smooth and uneventful. Mom and I had to cover a good deal of ground when we changed planes in Minneapolis. Fortunately, the medical staff in Columbus had arranged for me to have a wheelchair at Minneapolis, and we made our plane without incident and headed for Sioux Falls.

The streetlights in Sioux Falls shimmered from the heat of that August night when we touched down in the city around eleven. Dad picked us up at the airport in our black Honda Accord. He quickly loaded our luggage into the car, helped me into the front seat, and headed for Avera McKennan Hospital. Dad tried to talk to me during the brief drive, but because of my intense pain, I was less than receptive.

"So, did you make it to any car dealerships while you were in Columbus?" he asked.

"Yeah."

"OK, well, how about drum shops? I remember you always liked to go to drum shops there," he said.

"Yes."

"Oh, uh-huh. That's good. Where did you go?" he inquired.

"Dad, I'm sorry, but I don't really feel like talking right now. Just get me there," I implored. Dad shifted his focus to the streets and drove.

When we arrived at the emergency room, a couple of EMTs emerged from the hospital, loaded me into a wheelchair, and wheeled me into an examination room. A nurse came in and asked me to relate my story. We spent about fifteen minutes talking, and then I was taken up to a room in 3 East, which is where the hospital houses its cancer patients. Before giving me some pain medication, the nurse told me that Dr. Robert Nelimark would be my oncologist, and I would undergo a bone marrow biopsy the following morning. She tried to explain the procedure to me, but when she saw how exhausted I was, she left me to rest. The nurse turned out the light and let me try to sleep. The following day would be another big one.

My God, I thought to myself, *what have I gotten myself into?* I settled into the darkness of a dreamless sleep.

6

The Journey to Health Begins

I awoke in pain the following morning. Although my right leg still throbbed, I couldn't help but feel gratitude. For perhaps the first time in my life, I was truly grateful for another day, another sunrise. Waking up and seeing the light of a new day was something I had taken for granted the previous twenty years. Not that day.

A few hours later, a nurse came to my room and told me I would have a bone marrow biopsy that afternoon.

Oh, yeah … the bone marrow biopsy, I thought. I had forgotten about it in the confusion of the previous eight hours.

The nurse explained that the biopsy would involve penetrating one of my pelvis's iliac crests with a needle and aspirating a sample of bone marrow. The procedure would take only about fifteen minutes.

"Is it going to hurt?" I asked.

She said there would be some discomfort but assured me that lidocaine would be applied to the skin and bone. I understood that it would numb the skin where I would be stuck with the needle, but I didn't get how it would numb the bone. I didn't realize that the surface of bones had feeling. I learned in the hours that followed just how many nerves are in bone.

Around three, Nelimark came through my door; two nurses followed. He rehashed what the nurse had explained and asked me to lie on my stomach. Nelimark said the first step would be to apply the lidocaine.

When I had gotten Novocain shots in my gums, I had felt the needle prick for a moment and then sweet numbness soon followed. The lidocaine injection was a different story. Instead of a pinprick followed by a numbing sensation, the lidocaine burned as it entered my skin. The burning lasted for only a few seconds, but it was intense. I had never felt burning like that.

"Maybe this won't be so bad," I murmured. Little did I know.

Once my skin was numbed, it was time for the nurse to numb my iliac crest. The skin at the injection site had lost feeling, so I didn't feel pain when the needle penetrated my skin. But when the needle hit the bone, it definitely hurt. I'd never been pricked in rapid succession by the needle of a sewing machine, but I can imagine that the sensation would be similar. The pain, which felt like more burning or an electric shock, didn't last very long. But it certainly got my attention. Mild sedation would have been nice at that point, but I don't recall receiving any. That would change during bone marrow biopsies in the years that followed.

Nelimark and the attending nurses allowed the lidocaine a few minutes to fully take effect. When it did, Nelimark asked me to lie on my belly and tilt my body over to one side. I complied, and one of the nurses took my hand in hers. At first I thought the gesture was meant only to comfort me. And it was—no question about that. But I soon realized that the nurse's hand would give me something to squeeze during the procedure. It was a good thing, too. With each of the aspiration needle's pokes and prods into my iliac crest, I squeezed her hand tighter and tighter. In reality, I probably wasn't squeezing her hand all that hard, but there were times when the pain of the needle penetrating my bone was so intense that I felt I could have crushed her hand. With the procedure completed, Nelimark and the nurses left me alone. During those few hours, I watched some TV and tried to relax.

Around ten in the evening, I lay in the darkness of my room and tried to sleep. The nurses had given me some medication, but it wasn't doing much good. The pain I experienced in my leg, as well as in my right shoulder, was too great. Trying to sleep was futile. Still, I was used to sleeping and resting at night, so I tried to make myself go to sleep.

In a daze, I noticed that a shaft of light from the 3 East hallway soon cut through the darkness of the hospital room. I turned to face the light but found the pain surging through my right shoulder was too great. I couldn't see who was approaching, but a familiar voice soon let me know who had come to visit.

"Louis? Louis, are you all right?" said the voice that traveled my way from the light of the hallway.

It was my friend Nicomas and her companion, Art, whom I had gotten to know during my days at SDSU. They had driven more than fifty miles from their home in Brookings to see me. Unfortunately, I wasn't very good company.

"Nicomas, I hurt … I hurt my shoulder," was all I could utter.

"Oh, your shoulder hurts?" Nicomas asked. I replied in the affirmative. Taking that into consideration and noticing the time, Nicomas and Art excused themselves and headed back home. To this day, I feel bad for them, driving all that way to Sioux Falls to see me, and I wasn't able to make the visit worth their while. Still, the visit meant a lot to me. In a strange and alien place like a hospital, a friendly face is always welcome, regardless of how brief the visit.

7

Induction Chemotherapy

Fewer than forty-eight hours passed before the results of the bone marrow biopsy came back. I did have leukemia, as the doctor in Columbus had suspected. I had acute myeloid (or myelogenous) leukemia, or AML for short. Various forms of leukemia are identified and named based upon whether they are acute or chronic and upon the type of white blood cell that is affected.

Nelimark delivered the diagnosis. He also informed me that I was going to receive a regimen of chemotherapy in the hopes of putting me into a durable remission. Such treatments are called induction chemotherapy. In my case, the chemo would be a combination of two drugs: Ara-C and Idarubicin. The Ara-C would be delivered intravenously twenty-four hours a day for seven days. I would receive Idarubicin for twenty-four hours a day for three days. Nelimark told me a Hickman catheter would be installed in the right side of my chest. The catheter would have two ports dangling from the insertion point to allow chemotherapy, other medications, and blood products to be infused directly into my circulatory system. The end of the catheter inside my body would extend into my subclavian vein delivering whatever was infused into my superior vena cava. Any infused products would then be sent throughout my body courtesy of the pumping power of my heart. The catheter was installed that day, and I began chemotherapy within twenty-four hours.

Before the doctor left that day, I asked him what caused the leukemia. He said he didn't have a conclusive answer, but postulated that it was probably caused by something in the environment. I asked whether the illness could have been hereditary, and he told me it wasn't. He said it could have been caused by exposure to chemicals or to high doses of radiation. All I knew at the time was that I had a long road to recovery ahead of me; I didn't know how long and how hard that road would be.

Over the next seven days and beyond, about all I could was remain in my room and watch TV or don a blue surgical mask and walk the halls of McKennan's third floor. There were times I gratefully entertained visitors. I didn't start experiencing side effects from the Ara-C and Idarubicin infusions for a few days.

When I walked the corridor that connects 3 East and 3 West, I paused to look out the windows to the east. Prior to seeing eastern Sioux Falls from such a vantage point, I had never really noticed the green, rolling hills and ovular water towers. I vowed to myself that if I were ever able to do so again, I would explore those hilly regions and see what was there. I needed something to which I could cling, some tentative plan for the future.

One of the services available to McKennan patients was access to the hospital's extensive video library. Upon request, a nurse would retrieve requested videos and wheel a cart with a television and VCR into the room. Videos could be checked out for three days. My first selections were *Batman*; *1492: Conquest of Paradise*; and *Coneheads*. I took some pleasure in watching *Coneheads*, but perhaps the first two movies were not good choices.

It may have been the anxieties I was feeling about the possibility of being cooped up in the hospital for at least a month, but I found *Batman* difficult to watch. I had seen the movie several times on video since I first saw it with my childhood friend Ben in 1989, and the movie had never bothered me before. It may have had something to do with the film's dark themes and the acts of violence; I don't know. I do know that I didn't enjoy watching *Batman* at all.

While *Batman* disturbed me, nothing could have prepared me for how awful, how *angry* I felt watching the movie about Christopher Columbus. Don't get me wrong; the film had a lot of production value with good acting and beautiful cinematography. But the subject matter, which addressed Columbus's landing in the West Indies in 1492 and the subsequent slaughtering of the area's indigenous people, upset me to the core. Again, the agitation I experienced could be attributed to my circumstances, but if I were to watch the movie again, I'd likely experience the same reaction.

Before chemotherapy began, Nelimark and several nurses had described various side effects that I might experience from the drugs. Not all of them surfaced, but many did. Of those that did, not all surfaced immediately.

The most obvious side effect was nausea. There were times when I spontaneously got sick and vomited. But more often than not, vomiting followed eating or drinking. And there were times when even the mere scent of food trays as they were wheeled down the hospital hallways would cause me to retch. I would never call retching fun, and it was painful in many instances.

Speaking of pain, a side effect I endured during my first round of chemotherapy (but curiously and thankfully not during subsequent rounds) was mouth sores. The sores, open wounds on my gums, were generally unpleasant and especially painful when I tried to eat. Often I was unable to brush my teeth because feeling the prickly bristles against my gums made me want to climb the walls. Thankfully, the nurses proposed a solution. It wasn't a perfect solution, but it worked for the time

I needed it. The nurses instructed me to dab a mouth swab with tooth-paste and clean my teeth and gums with it.

My hair, which I had cropped several weeks before, stayed firmly attached to my head until the day before I was released from the hospital on September 9. With each successive round of chemo, my hair usually fell out within twenty-four hours. In the first case, however, it held out for about three weeks. There was even a time when Nelimark wondered if perhaps I would be one of the few people who managed to keep his hair. But less than a day after Nelimark posed the question, my hair fell out. And it wasn't just the hair on my head; all the hair on my body except my eyebrows fell out.

Side effects weren't the main concerns that Nelimark and I had regarding the chemotherapy. The chief concern was whether the treatment would work. Nelimark told me that the only way to find out would be to perform another bone marrow biopsy. But that couldn't be done until ten days after chemotherapy. Between the end of chemo and the bone marrow biopsy, the minutes, hours, and days crawled by. I practically counted the minutes. My desire to leave that hospital and return to my "normal," healthy life was strong.

Visitors came and went during my first round of chemotherapy and during the following weeks when my immune system was recovering from the chemical assault. Among them were coworkers, including our director and Jim, and old high school friends like Brian, Jeff, David, and Stac; Valerian visited me a few times as well. But the people who were with me every day were my parents. Regardless of how out-of-it I felt or how down I was, Mom and Dad were always there. Each day Dad drove to Colman, South Dakota, to pick up Mom from work, and the two headed to the hospital to spend about an hour with me. If Mom and Dad, along with everyone else who came out of the wood-work and supported me, had not been there with me to buoy my spirits, I'm sure the outcome of the chemo and the leukemia would have been very different. They all were the foundation to which I anchored myself. I certainly didn't want to die, but the thought of leaving people whom I loved dearly was too painful and daunting to me to allow myself to give up the fight.

No one who visited me ever showed signs of being upset with me and my situation, but one person who called did express a great deal of emotion. One afternoon during my first week of chemo, I received a phone call from a friend in Rapid City. He was a relative of a good friend of mine, and I had come to know him and his family a few winters prior.

When he called, he wanted to know how I was feeling; I wanted to know the same about him. He seemed kind of reserved on the phone, as though he was searching for the words to say to me. Perhaps they would have been words of comfort or encouragement. We exchanged a few words, and nausea kicked in. I excused myself from the phone for a moment to vomit. When I finished, I picked up the receiver and asked for my friend's pardon. My request was met with sobs; he couldn't continue and hung up. I realized how much what was happening to me impacted the people in my life. And I regretted that my illness brought sadness and worry to those close to me. Knowing that my survival would restore some peace to the lives of my loved ones motivated me to not give up. I didn't want to die and leave those I cared about behind. It was then that I decided to work and fight as hard as I could to beat the disease. I didn't really know how to win my fight but was determined to struggle against the leukemia regardless.

8

Praying for a Good Outcome

Hours and days crawled by—or at least seemed to—between the end of my chemotherapy and the time I would have another bone marrow biopsy. I occupied myself with lots of television (mostly music videos on VH1), sleep when I could fall into it, and company who visited. I thought about having to spend lots of time in the hospital. It was strange; the thought of dying wasn't something that really concerned me at that point. I was more concerned about dealing with the discomfort and ennui of having to spend perhaps months at a time in a hospital room.

The night before the bone marrow biopsy was to occur, I took my usual evening stroll around 3 East. I had plenty of energy, but being strapped to an IV pole impeded my movements. As I walked around the nurses' station with the IV pole in tow, I noticed the chapel on one side of the hallway. I don't know why, but I felt the need to go into that chapel that night and pray for a good outcome for the bone marrow biopsy. There was no reason I couldn't have prayed from my hospital room, but going into the chapel seemed appropriate. No one else was using it, so I made myself as comfortable as I could, knelt, and began to entreat the Creator for good health and for a life beyond that night. When I left the chapel that evening, I didn't have any overwhelming sense that everything would be all right. But I did feel content that I had said my piece.

Hours later, after the dawn had come and gone, Nelimark and a team of nurses interrupted my TV watching to do the bone marrow biopsy. The experience wasn't unlike my first bone marrow biopsy. Nelimark asked me to lie face down on the bed. He then administered some local anesthetic to the site from which the bone marrow sample would be aspirated. This biopsy was performed on the opposite side of my pelvis. Nelimark said he doesn't like to perform successive biopsies on the same site.

Nelimark numbed the skin and the bone at the aspiration site. Once again, I clenched my paled fingers around those of a nurse. Nelimark didn't seem to have too much trouble driving the thick needle through the skin and muscle in my lower back. And it didn't take him too long to prod the tip of the needle through the surface bone on my iliac crest. I never would have known the relative ease with which he was performing his task, though. I was in as much pain as I was during the first biopsy. Tiny shocks of agony shot through my entire system each time the needle's tip attempted to penetrate my bone. Thankfully, the procedure lasted no more than about fifteen minutes, and the pain subsided quickly once the needle was withdrawn. A nurse, seeing that I was perspiring through the pain, wet a rag and dabbed my forehead. I thanked her for her assistance and was once again left alone to go back to my TV watching. There was nothing left to do besides wait, watch TV, and pray. The results wouldn't come for another twenty-four hours.

Twenty-four hours came and went, as did three meals that I could barely eat. Eating was especially laborious, not only because of nausea, but because of the sores that had developed in my mouth. The fact that the odor of hospital cafeteria fare sickened me didn't help, either.

By five in the afternoon, Mom had gotten off work and Dad had stopped at Colman to pick her up and bring her to McKennan. Around that time, Nelimark had some news to share with all of us. Mom, Dad, and I waited nervously to hear the results of the latest bone marrow biopsy. Much to our relief, Nelimark told us that the test had shown that the leukemia had gone into remission, and that the only thing standing between me and getting out of the hospital was my white blood cell count. Once my white blood cell count, particularly my neutrophils, rose above a certain level, my immune system would be strong enough to allow me to survive outside the protective environment of 3 East.

Release from the hospital came about a week later. My stay in McKennan, from the time I was admitted after arriving from Columbus to being released on September 9, was about three and a half weeks. That first stay would prove to be one of the shortest spans I would spend in the hospital over the next nine months.

My release couldn't have come soon enough. Getting out on September 9 turned out to be a happy coincidence. I knew that the first Native American Club gathering of the academic year was going to be held that evening, and I wanted to attend if I were healthy enough. That day also turned out to be the day that my eight-inch Premier XPK tom-tom arrived from Interstate Musician Supply. I had ordered the component drum with the idea of making the set of Premier drums that I purchased in November 1998 a seven-piece drum kit. After I got home from the hospital, I examined and tuned the drum before I went to the Native American Club picnic.

I don't recall there being that many native students attending the picnic, but there were several members of SDSU's faculty there, including Velva-Lu, the university's Native American student adviser. Everyone seemed to be well aware of the health crisis I was facing, and everyone expressed great concern about my overall health. They seemed pleased to see me out of the hospital, and it was good to be among people again and to eat real food. Unfortunately, I still wasn't able to enjoy the food much because of the nausea and the mouth sores. But at least it wasn't hospital food.

In the week that followed, I visited Nelimark in Sioux Falls. During our office visit, he told me that the next step in my treatment would be to travel to the Mayo Clinic in Rochester, Minnesota, to consult with a hematologist. I never fully learned why it was so important that I see the hematologist, but I suppose that he was somebody whom Nelimark believed was very competent. An appointment was set up for a few weeks later, and during that visit, the hematologist would lay out the remainder of my treatment. That's assuming, of course, that I would survive.

Between my exit from McKennan and my visit to the Mayo Clinic, I tried to return to the normalcy of my life in whatever ways possible. I was in no condition yet to take classes at SDSU, and it would have been difficult to enroll because the semester had already started. Besides, Nelimark and others advised me to rest.

Although I couldn't effectively get back into the swing of things in school, I did resolve to go back to work in the FacLab as soon as I felt able. In fact, I went back to work a few days after getting out of McKennan. Keeping myself occupied turned out to be a good idea, but it was a somewhat difficult transition from sitting in a hospital room for days on end to going back to working part-time at the university. I felt fine physically for the most part. I was self-conscious, however, about losing my hair. My hair had not completely fallen out, and what hair remained tended to fall out in clumps throughout the days following my release from McKennan. The first few days I went back to work, I wore a ball cap to try to conceal the alopecia as best I could. Before too long, however, I decided that I didn't like wearing the ball cap (I was never much of a hat wearer), so I went to my friend Jan and asked her to shave off what hair I had left. It took a few days for me to adjust to the thought of being bald, but I got used to being a chrome dome rather quickly. Not having hair became a nonissue for me, and I no longer dreaded looking at myself in the mirror and seeing a pale, thin, hairless reflection of myself.

Life during the days after McKennan wasn't too bad. I often felt weak and had to be on guard for nausea, but things could have been worse. Over time, my mouth sores began to heal, and my energy level began to return. My energy level never fully recovered until many months later, but I managed to gather enough strength to go out among people and function as normally as possible.

My days were pretty good, but nights were rough. Life for me has always been more difficult in the night than in the daytime, but battling cancer made the nights that much more laborious. There were nights on end when I would go to bed around seven in the evening because I was too tired to do anything else but wouldn't fall asleep for at least three hours. Many evenings, in the soft light of the setting sun, I would alternately watch TV and toss and turn, hoping for sleep to come. With all of the tossing and turning, I felt a great deal of anxiety over lying on my Hickman catheter and pulling it out of my chest. I never did "lie wrong" or pull the catheter out of my chest, but the plastic tubing dangling from the right side of my chest always represented a concern.

When I finally settled into sleep, I didn't dream all that much. There were a few times, however, when the dreams that I had would be quite vivid and lifelike. In all of the dreams I remember, I saw myself. And when I saw myself, it was as though I perceived the action in the dream from two perspectives. Sometimes I would observe my environment in the dream state from a usual first-person perspective. That is, I witnessed the events in my dreams through my own eyes. Other times, I saw other characters in the dreams, as well as myself, from a third-person perspective. I was experiencing the dream as if I were watching a TV show or a movie.

When I saw myself from a third-person perspective, my concept of myself was always the same: I would rarely see my face in the dream but would often see myself from behind, as though looking at myself and people with whom I was interacting through the lens of a camera mounted behind me at a forty-five-degree angle. And when I would see myself, I would always appear to be healthy; I had a full head of hair, albeit longer than the cropped coif I commonly wore at the time. And judging by the way I carried myself, I stood tall and healthy.

9

Visit to the Mayo Clinic

In early October, Mom, Dad, and I packed up the car to head to the Mayo Clinic. None of us really knew what to expect at the world-renowned Rochester, Minnesota, medical facility. What we did know, though, was that we would need to be there for two days for tests and to see the doctor.

Until that time, I spent my days assisting faculty members in the FacLab when I felt strong enough to do so, and I putzed around the house with Dad while Mom worked. Every few weeks, I attended Native American Club meetings. In spite of my sickness, I had been elected secretary/treasurer of the Native American Club. And having that added responsibility, along with my work with the Instructional Technologies Center, helped me stay strong and look forward to each coming day. Having places to go, people to see, and things to do helped keep me anchored to the day-to-day world to which I desperately yearned to return.

When I had accepted the nomination for secretary/treasurer of the Native American Club, many in the club raised concerns about my ability to fulfill my duties. They were merely looking out for my well-being. I assured them that I felt up to holding such an office and per-forming the duties attached to it, so the group elected me. It turned out that I missed few meetings in spite of being in the hospital so much in the following few months. I did miss the powwow while I was in the hospital, but everyone seemed pleased that I was able to contribute to the group's efforts whenever I could.

The day to head to the Mayo Clinic finally came. I don't remember much about the day, apart from the fact that the drive was about 250 miles, and it was sunny and fairly warm for October. I didn't feel like driving, so Mom and Dad handled wheel duties. We left Aurora early in the morning and arrived in Rochester in the early afternoon. We stopped for a quick bite to eat and then stopped at Best Buy so I could check out what music was available.

We hadn't made reservations for some reason, and we didn't find a motel right away. Instead we went directly to the Mayo Clinic so that I could check in and register for tests and the doctor visit the next day.

Finding a motel turned out to be something of a struggle. None of us knew Rochester very well, and none of us thought to pick up a road map. We finally found a cheap little place on one of the city's main drags, not far from the hospital. The place looked rather low-rent, but each room was laid out like an efficiency apartment. The room had the feel of a living room, with two twin-size beds on one side of the room and a television on the other about twenty feet away. Between the bed and the TV was a recliner chair, where I spent a good deal of time when I wasn't in the clinic. Mom and Dad were ready to crash by the time we checked into the room, but I didn't feel ready to sleep yet. My dog-eared copy of James Welch's *Fools Crow* kept me company. I've loved that book since I first read it, and I still consider it one of my favorite books of all time. I've always appreciated the detail and the humanity with which Welch imbued his characters, and I've enjoyed exploring what life is like for various groups of people at different points in history.

The next morning, I didn't feel especially nervous upon rising from a dreamless sleep, but I didn't feel great either. I can't imagine that anyone feels good having to travel hundreds of miles to receive news regarding an uncertain future. The feeling was probably similar to facing the county hangman in years past. At least the nurses were nice while they took blood samples and ran me through MRIs. Nothing could have prepared me, though, for what happened when I saw the doctor.

My appointment with the hematologist was scheduled for around three in the afternoon. Mom, Dad, and I stepped off the elevator at the appropriate floor and took seats near the entrance to the corridor where the examining rooms were. The appointed time came and went, and then another hour, and then another hour. Three hours after we arrived, my name was finally called. With a sense of relief and frustration, I slinked over to the nurse. But I was feeling some trepidation, too, for what lay waiting for me beyond the door. Over the past three hours, most of the patients, especially the women, who emerged from the examining rooms and doctor consultations, were in tears. Crying usually isn't a good sign, especially when one's life may hang in the balance.

Another kind nurse led me to a small room, the centerpiece of which was a black examining table. There was nothing noteworthy about the room, but there was at least a window out of which I could see the sun nearing the end of its journey to the horizon. She took my vitals, jotted down a few notes, and asked me to get undressed for the doctor's examination. The nurse left, and I complied with her request. I wasn't provided with a gown or any kind of sheet; at that point modesty wasn't the first thing on my mind.

With my jeans, T-shirt, socks, and shoes resting together in a pile in a corner of the room, I took my place on one end of the examining table. There wasn't anything to do but sit, wait, and hope for the best. There weren't any magazines in the room, and everything was awash in cold black and silver. The room looked modern, not at all warm and inviting.

After about ten minutes, the hematologist knocked on the door and entered. He introduced himself, shook my hand, and got down to business. He seemed pleasant enough, but I didn't feel at ease around him. Then again, I suppose it's hard for anyone to feel at ease when he's sitting stark naked on a cold examining table under the scrutiny of a complete stranger.

He circled me a few times, saying nothing. He spoke no words but communicated through his stony expression. It's not as though I expected him to be grinning and cheerful. But I didn't expect him to be so cold and clinical. He shined lights into my eyes, ears, and mouth, and occasionally poked and prodded my torso. After circling me a few times, he threw a stony glance down to my lower torso, and then his eyes met mine.

"Are you keeping your penis clean?" he said.

His question was legitimate, I suppose, but I didn't see what it had to do with my leukemia. Perhaps it did, but as far as I could see, it didn't. I can only guess that he noted that I'm uncircumcised and wondered if my personal hygiene extended to my genitals. I answered that yes, I kept my penis clean, and the conversation ended there. The doctor, whose mid-thirties face hadn't softened from a scowl, told me I could get dressed. He said he was going to step out for a few minutes and would return to discuss the remainder of my treatment. The lone gesture of kindness he extended to me was asking if I wanted my parents in the room with us when he would lay the news on me. I replied in the affirmative, and a nurse fetched Mom and Dad.

By the time Mom and Dad took chairs next to mine, I didn't feel very well. I felt weak and tired from all of the drama and anticipation. Both tried to reassure me that everything would be all right, and I wanted so desperately to believe them. But it was out of our hands at that point.

The hematologist returned, planted himself firmly on the four-legged, wheeled stool, introduced himself to Mom and Dad, and then glanced over his notes for a moment. He began outlining what my overall condition was. He didn't say that my situation was grave, but he did say there was still a long road ahead. I was in remission, but a number of steps would be required to keep me in a durable remission. Since the discussion during the next several minutes would likely have serious bearings on the direction of the remainder of my life, we hung on the doctor's every word. And it was that hanging on every word that made what happened next especially difficult.

Two or three times, just as the hematologist got to a critical point in the conversation—usually related to whether I would need a bone marrow transplant and more chemotherapy and my chances of survival—his pager went off. He glanced down at it and excused himself to make a phone call. His callousness created crushing suspense for my parents and me. I had never had such a sense of impending doom.

My God ... what's going to happen? I kept thinking to myself. And I have no doubt the same thought ran through my parents' minds, too.

When the doctor finally decided to give us his undivided attention, he sat down and laid before us the "options" available. I was in tears by that point, but choked them back enough to compose myself to continue the discussion with the doctor.

He said the ultimate solution for me would be to have a bone marrow transplant. Given the information he had, the chances of dying from the transplant were 25 percent. Such a percentage was small, but not small enough to be trivial, he said. The best thing to do from that point was to undergo the same regimen of chemotherapy that I had had when I was first put into remission. Once that was finished and I had sufficiently recovered, I would have outpatient chemotherapy for four or five months. We visited for a few minutes more, and then Mom,

Dad, and I quietly left the office as so many others had that day—in tears. The news we received wasn't terrible, but it wasn't great either. At least hope was still alive.

The mid-October daylight was failing fast by the time we reached the car and prepared for what lay ahead. We didn't have a room reservation for the night, so we decided to take advantage of the remaining good weather and head back to Brookings. We stopped for a quick bite to eat. Mom and Dad didn't eat much; they each picked up a hamburger at McDonald's, and I had a Big Mac. It was good to eat again after having waited for so long in the doctor's office. But the circumstances of our situation and the dread of not knowing what was in store sucked much of the flavor out of the food. And to top it all off, a mild tooth discomfort in one of my upper molars began to develop as we cruised west on Interstate 90 toward Sioux Falls. One of my worst fears had been realized: I was starting to have dental problems, and there was little I could do about it. My highest thoughts were on simple survival, on keeping alive. But I spent a lot of my time on the trip home to Brookings that night hoping that at least my pained tooth could be addressed.

We arrived in Brookings around one the following morning. None of us slept well that night, especially Mom. And she had to get up and go to work that day, so it was stressful for her. I didn't have anything pressing going on that morning, apart from getting in touch with Nelimark to see if my immune system would be strong enough to have my teeth checked.

10

Tooth Trouble

In the mid-morning hours of the day following our return from the Mayo Clinic, I was able to get in touch with Nelimark to ask him if I could see a dentist. He said that my immune system was likely strong enough. But he also said it would be wise to start taking an antibiotic to help deal with any possible infections. We also discussed plans for starting my second round of chemotherapy. Nelimark and I scheduled my return to the hospital for a few weeks from that time, which gave me some time to get my teeth fixed.

When I finished talking to Nelimark, I contacted various dentists around town. It turns out that only one could take me on as a patient and do the work required. I made an appointment to see the dentist a few days later.

In the meantime, the pain I was experiencing had subsided some, but the thought of having a major toothache continued to resonate through my mind. To keep my mind off such things, I put in as much time at ITC as I could and kept in touch with friends. A group of my friends, sensing the disturbance of my peace of mind, took me out one night and tried to give me a good time. We shot pool and hung out, and being surrounded by friends helped. But in my heart, I knew that only a visit to the dentist could deal with what was on my mind.

The following day, I decided to work on a design for the Native American Club's 2000 powwow poster. My dentist appointment wasn't until the afternoon, so I had some time. I had never designed a powwow poster before, but I had tools at my disposal that I could use. Those tools included the Adobe PageMaker software, as well as the skills I had gained from taking a typography course the previous semester. I didn't get the entire design done before heading off to see the dentist, but I accomplished a fair bit of work done. Having the image that our NAC president had drawn helped. I used it as the basis for the design.

Since I still felt pretty weak, I asked Dad to drive me to the dentist; he was happy to oblige. After we arrived, the hygienist took me to one of the dental chairs and captured some images on X-ray film. The dentist then came in and consulted with me and took a look inside my mouth. The source of my discomfort was readily apparent to him; one of my wisdom teeth was "rotting" and needed to be removed. I found the idea of having a tooth removed somewhat unsettling, given the fact that I'd never had a tooth removed and wasn't a fan of having dental work done. Still, I readily consented, knowing that the tooth removal would relieve my pain. I scheduled an appointment for the following day.

A day later, Dad drove me back to the dentist's office to have the tooth extracted. As is natural, I was filled with trepidation regarding the pain I might experience both during and after the procedure. The hygienist sensed my concern and suggested that I might want some nitrous oxide gas to take the edge off. I thought that was a good idea, and she placed a gas mask over my nose and gave me a dose of the gas as the dentist started injecting Novocain into the gum tissue surrounding the tooth that would be removed. The nitrous oxide didn't have quite as acute an effect as I had expected, but I sensed that it caused some sensation changes for me. Mainly I noticed that my lower extremities became tingly.

After about five minutes, my gums were well-numbed. Then the dentist inserted an instrument that must have resembled pliers into my mouth. Fearing the worst, I found myself tensing up and expecting to feel a lot of pain. To my surprise, there was no pain. I could feel pressure, and I could feel the dentist working the rotting molar side to side in my jaw, but there was no pain. It didn't take long for the dentist to wrest the tooth from my mouth and tidy up, and I was grateful for that. I was most grateful, however, because the experience hadn't been anywhere near as painful as I had expected. There was still concern regarding how much pain I might feel once the Novocain lost its potency. But at least the procedure was over, and the source of my dental pain had been excised. The dentist gave me a prescription for Tylenol with codeine and sent me on my way. Dad took me back home so I could rest, and he went to the store to fill the prescription. My recovery seemed to take only a few days, and I was grateful for that. The greatest blessing was my toothache was gone. At least I could face the future without having to worry about my teeth.

In the few weeks that followed before I reentered the hospital, I continued to work at ITC when I was able to assist faculty members with their educational technology projects. The interaction with others, particularly with those who were aware of my situation and who expressed their concern, was good. Being among other people helped me maintain at least some semblance of normalcy when life itself had been effectively turned upside down. Apart from work, I took care of what Native American Club business I could and spent time with friends. There were also visits with Nelimark a few times a week, as well as a few blood transfusions. Fortunately, it worked out that most of the blood transfusions were coupled with doctor visits, so Mom, Dad, and I wouldn't have to make as many trips to Sioux Falls as we would otherwise.

I found that blood transfusions weren't all that unpleasant, but they were time-consuming. For me, they turned out to be among those experiences that seem agonizingly slow when one is undertaking them but aren't so bad when looked upon in hindsight. Each unit of blood required about four hours to fully transfuse, and most of the transfusions were given in a large room in which others were also being transfused. The room was filled with comfortable leather recliners and TVs mounted on flexible stands. There were also larger television screens mounted near the ceiling. Before each transfusion began, some intravenous Benadryl was injected into one of the ports of my Hickman catheter. I imagine that the antihistamine was to prevent any allergic reactions to the blood products, regardless of whether they were red blood cells or platelets. Whatever the Benadryl was for, it made me sleepy. And it was that sleepiness that allowed me to slumber through much of the transfusion process. Sleeping through a transfusion occurred most frequently in the rare instances when I was transfused while lying in a hospital bed.

It was after one such transfusion when concern arose that I would need another transfusion to replace the blood that I had already received. Late one evening, after returning from Avera McKennan, I walked into the house from the garage and made my way to the living room of the Aurora farmhouse. Before leaving for Sioux Falls, I had left a pair of shoes lying on the floor. I tripped over the shoes and fell in such a way that my nose hit one of the living room walls. Mom and Dad picked me up off the floor, and my nose began to bleed. At first we wondered if I would need to return to Sioux Falls to have another transfusion. The bleeding was controlled before too long, however, and I didn't lose much blood. At that point, I hoped I wouldn't need to make any other trips to the hospital and receive additional transfusions until I had to return to the hospital for more chemotherapy.

During the late afternoon hours of the day before my return to the hospital for more chemotherapy, my friends Chris and Aaron took me for a ride out to Oakwood Lakes. The early fall air was still fairly warm, but was chilly enough for me to need to wear a sweatshirt and jacket. During our visit to Oakwood Lakes, the three of us walked the Teton-kaha Trail on Boy Scout Island and did what hiking we could. It was really nice to be out in the fresh fall air, especially considering that none of us knew what the future had in store for me. For all we knew, I might never leave the hospital once I entered it. I never seriously entertained the thought that I could die in the hospital but did acknowledge that such an occurrence was a possibility. Something within me told me that I would survive, and being surrounded by so many friends and family buoyed my spirits through it all.

11

Chemo, Round 2

Mom, Dad, and I, as we had done so many times in the previous few months, made our way to Avera McKennan hospital. This trip would be different from prior trips, however. This time my parents would return home while I remained at the hospital.

Nelimark and a team of nurses admitted me to the hospital in the early afternoon, and by the middle of the afternoon I settled into my room. Rather than wait a day as I had when I entered the hospital as an inpatient the first time, I would begin chemotherapy right away. My treatment was scheduled to begin around eight that night. In the meantime, I did what I could to make myself comfortable and to ready myself for what I knew could be another long hospital stay.

The regimen of drugs I was to receive was the same as the one I had received when I underwent induction chemotherapy: seven days' worth of Ara-C and three days' worth of Idarubicin. In addition, I would be given other drugs as necessary to combat nausea and other forms of pain and discomfort.

Fluorescent light from the rig above the bed provided the only light in the room. On the TV was an image of Sylvester Stallone, as Rocky, trudging through the snow with a log on his back. It turns out that Spike TV or one of the other cable networks was showing a *Rocky* marathon that week, and I happened to catch part of *Rocky IV*.

My chemotherapy hadn't started by the time I was ready to sleep. The nurse came in to hook up the Ara-C and Idarubicin infusion around 9:30 PM. It took her only a few minutes to get everything up and running. I had no idea what side effects I could expect this time around or how long I would be in the hospital. But at least I knew the drill and had some firsthand experience with chemotherapy. Within the first few minutes of the infusion, I noticed that the infusion device was louder than I expected. The noise amounted to little more than a good deal of ticking, but the ticking was pronounced. I called the nurse, and she offered to drape a towel over the IV pole. The towel didn't quell the noise completely but seemed effective enough. The only time I noticed the noise was when I was awake. And I spent a lot of time awake in the following week.

The week that followed that night was similar to the week when I went through my first round of chemotherapy. One key difference was that I wasn't trying to get into remission; I was already in remission and was now trying to stay in remission. Another difference was that some of the side effects of the chemo were less severe, while others were more severe. One side effect that improved was mouth sores. I didn't have any mouth sores during the second round of chemotherapy or at any rounds after the first round of chemotherapy. I'm not sure why. My best guess is that the antibacterial toothpaste the dentist prescribed for me after the wisdom tooth removal helped.

Nausea, however, was particularly pronounced. I had experienced nausea before but never like I did during chemotherapy. And the nausea seemed the most severe after I ate or drank anything. There were several times when I would wake up thirsty in the middle of the night and would drink my fill of water. Minutes later, I'd have to call the nurse to help me clean up the mess from vomiting. Not being able to keep food or drink down had its consequences. I lost a lot of weight during and in the aftermath of the second chemotherapy. I still weighed over two hundred pounds when I entered the hospital in late October. I weighed about 155 in all of my hairless pallor when I left the hospital.

I spent roughly five weeks in the hospital in October and November of 1999, but those five weeks weren't contiguous. The first week was the time during which I underwent my second round of chemotherapy. During that week, I pleaded with Nelimark to let me go home after the chemotherapy if my blood counts were high enough. To my surprise, he consented. At the end of the week, my white blood cell counts were still at a relatively safe level, so Nelimark cut me loose and told me to rest at home. He said I should visit the Brookings Hospital daily and have blood counts checked; the counts would then be sent to Nelimark. Words couldn't describe how good I felt when I was told that I could leave the hospital after spending a week there.

I was filled with another good feeling when Nelimark visited me one night in the middle of the week of chemotherapy. Nelimark performed another bone marrow biopsy to get a feel for the overall status of my bone marrow. He reported that there was no sign of leukemia in the marrow. And he said that when he checked the marrow down to the chromosomal level, there were no signs of the kind of abnormality that supposedly caused the leukemia. I didn't fully understand what Nelimark meant when he was talking about chromosomal abnormalities. But I knew that Nelimark's revelation was a good sign. I asked Nelimark what the abnormality was and what may have caused it. He said that in my case, the anomaly occurred when a piece of one of my chromosomes broke apart and attached itself to another of my chromosomes. And that attachment caused a chain reaction of genetic mutations that led to my marrow going astray. As for the cause of the abnormality, Nelimark really couldn't say. He postulated that the cause could have been something environmental such as exposure to chemicals or being struck by a burst of radiation.

As per the doctor's orders, I spent the following days at home, except for my daily visits to the Brookings Hospital. My blood counts remained above the required level, but I didn't feel very well as I began the recovery from the chemotherapy. Within five days after I was released from McKennan Hospital, I found myself once again within the confines of 3 East. At least the scenery changed a bit; I was in a different room.

In the week when I was home from the hospital, I picked up a staph infection. A staph infection is serious under any circumstance, but is especially dangerous for someone with virtually no functional immune system. I probably should have died from the infection. At Nelimark's insistence, I entered McKennan once more, and there I remained until after Thanksgiving.

During the following four weeks, I had to recover from the one-two punches I had been dealt. I needed to heal from the chemotherapy coupled with the staph infection. Unfortunately, there was little I could do apart from try to remain positive and rest. The remainder of my recovery was up to Nelimark and others charged with my care. My parents and friends like Chris and Valerian played key roles as well. Having Mom and Dad at my side at least once a day and being visited by others who cared strengthened my resolve. I'm not sure how close to death I was during that time. I do know that I wanted to fight as hard as necessary to keep from being separated from those I loved.

Over the course of four weeks, I received IV doses of various antibiotics employed to combat the infection. I also received antinausea medication so I could keep my food and drink down better. The medication prevented nausea but did little to help my appetite. It's kind of funny—when one hasn't eaten for several days, one stops feeling hungry. Though I hardly ate much of anything in those four weeks in the hospital, I was spared the usual pangs of hunger. Saline solution delivered via IV was my constant companion.

Another medication with which I became acquainted during the hospital stay was morphine. I didn't receive much morphine, but I experienced enough to know that it provided some relief from both the physical pain and the ennui of being confined to a hospital bed for days on end. Morphine was first given to me to alleviate some abdominal pain. The source of the pain was never pinpointed, but morphine took the pain away.

When I received my first four milligrams of morphine, the experience was unlike any I had had before. The nurse infused the drug into my Hickman catheter over the course of about ten seconds. And then a few seconds after that, I felt a burning sensation that seemed to radiate out from my core down my arms and legs. The burning wasn't altogether intense, but it felt like my innards were on fire. Not long after, the burning sensation gave way to an overwhelming sense of calm and relaxation. Any pain that I felt disappeared. I received a lot of morphine injections in the following weeks. And it was during that time that I became concerned about the possibility of developing an addiction to morphine. No addiction developed, however.

Despite the bleakness of my situation and condition, things started to look up after the first couple of weeks in the hospital. My blood counts began to creep upward, and I had my share of visitors. In the meantime, some strange physical problems began happening. First, the whites of my eyes became blood red. Nelimark and the nurses explained to me that the chemotherapy I had received had caused the blood vessels on the surface of my eyes to rupture. Fortunately, my eyes looked worse than they felt. My vision didn't seem to be affected, and the whites of my eyes returned to their normal color within a few weeks of my release.

Another physical problem was numbness in the pinkie of my right hand. Like the color of the whites of my eyes, the numbness and tingling were attributed to the chemotherapy. Also like the bloodiness of my eyes, the condition disappeared within a few weeks.

One ailment that still puzzles me is what some people call "chemo brain." Chemo brain was something I didn't realize I was experiencing until Valerian visited one night. He and I talked as we often did. But the conversation didn't flow as smoothly as it normally would. I found that I could form coherent thoughts in my mind, but I had greater difficulty than normal articulating my thoughts and feelings. My speech was slurred. Fortunately, Valerian and others who witnessed my slurred speech and other speaking difficulties understood the source of my condition. My normal speech patterns returned within a few weeks.

Since I wasn't released from the hospital until the end of November, I spent both my twenty-second birthday and Thanksgiving in the hospital. I didn't enjoy spending either occasion in the hospital. But at least I was able to spend time with loved ones during both times. I was showered with cards and gifts and was in touch with a lot of people during those dark times.

Regardless of what I missed by being in the hospital while recovering from chemotherapy and from the staph infection, I was grateful to once again be released. The order for my release was given midafternoon, but I wasn't wheeled out of the hospital until the light of day had already given way to the darkness of the late-fall evening. Since I hadn't had "real food" for more than a month, I asked Mom and Dad to run through the drive-through window at Arby's so I could get a roast beef and cheddar sandwich. Mom and Dad were happy to oblige, and with what little strength I had, I soon held the steaming sandwich in my hands. I took a bite, chewed, and savored the taste as best I could. Unfortunately, I realized that the chemotherapy had robbed me of some of my sense of taste. So I couldn't enjoy the sandwich as I normally would. Still, although I couldn't fully taste such food for a few weeks, I was happy to eat something other than hospital food. And although the future still remained a question mark, I felt happy to head home again and to know that I was hopefully on the home stretch for my cancer treatment.

12

Relapse

Life returned to some semblance of normalcy in the days and weeks that followed my release from the hospital. Slowly, my sense of taste returned, some color came back to my skin, and stubbly hair began to grow on my scalp. In the meantime, I continued to visit Nelimark in Sioux Falls a few times a week. Our visits largely consisted of blood draws and discussing my health. Strangely, we never set any plans for when my outpatient chemotherapy would begin. The Mayo Clinic hematologist had never indicated how much time should elapse between my inpatient chemo and my outpatient chemo, so I assumed it was up to Nelimark.

My birthday and Thanksgiving had come and gone, and Christmas was around the corner. As much as possible, Mom, Dad, and I prepared to celebrate the holiday season. In the meantime, I registered for classes for the spring 2000 semester. I knew I wouldn't have the energy or strength to carry my usually heavy course load. So I signed up for a few journalism classes, such as mass communication law, and an American Indian studies class taught by Valerian. It was hard to know what schedule to set since I didn't know the status of my chemotherapy, but I did the best that I could. I knew I would need to continue to visit McKennan a few times per week for blood work and for periodic transfusions.

Hours of daylight continued to get shorter as we descended into the depths of early winter, and then the days began to get a little longer as the spring semester began in early January. I was ready for classes.

Because I was still weak, it took me longer than usual to walk from class to class. Fortunately, my classes were spread far enough apart so I wouldn't have to rush. I was also lucky to find parking spaces close to the buildings in which I had classes.

I occupied myself outside of class with work at the FacLab and working with the Native American Club in getting ready for the powwow. Once the semester began, there were only about six weeks left before the powwow. And the club was in high gear making preparations. Most of the work involved planning and contacting vendors and officials who would be affiliated with the powwow. We also put on Indian taco sales and raffled off tickets for a star quilt to raise additional funds.

One cold, dark January morning, I spent about an hour in the basement of SDSU's Nursing, Family and Consumer Sciences, and Arts and Science building attending my mass communication law class. We had spent the first day of class going over the content of the class, and it was during the following class sessions that we discussed the early stages of American law.

I had another Nelimark checkup in late morning, so I had made arrangements to miss work that day so I could get checked. Everyone was so understanding about my work and my classes.

As was usual, Dad drove me to Avera McKennan for blood work. Afterward, Nelimark examined me before cutting me loose for the day. There was still no discussion about when my outpatient chemotherapy would begin, and I began to wonder what was going to happen. There didn't appear to be any immediate threat of recurrence of the leukemia, but I still was concerned about what lay ahead.

That afternoon, I returned home and spent some time resting and working on powwow stuff. A little more than an hour before Mom was to come home, I received a call from Nelimark. I initially thought that he was going to report that my blood results had come back and that everything continued to be all right.

"I really hate to tell you this, Lou," Nelimark began, "but it looks like the leukemia is coming back."

My first reaction wasn't shock. As I had reacted when I first learned that I had leukemia five months prior, I remained calm and asked Nelimark what needed to be done. I assumed that more chemo would be necessary, but I wanted to hear what Nelimark had to say. Nelimark asked me to meet him in Sioux Falls the next morning. In the meantime, I broke the news to Dad, and we both filled Mom in on what was happening once she returned home.

The following day, Mom, Dad, and I visited with Nelimark at McKennan. He told us that I would need more chemotherapy to put me back into remission. Nelimark said that because the leukemia had become resistant to some of the chemotherapeutic drugs, a different regimen would be used. Then he laid the really heavy news on us: the ultimate solution was a bone marrow transplant. None of us felt good about what was happening, and I certainly didn't like the prospect of going through the transplant—especially if it might mean having to stay in the hospital for more than a month. Again, it was strange that I didn't feel too concerned about dying; I was more concerned about getting through the treatment with my sanity and spirit intact.

I knew that returning to McKennan as an inpatient was inevitable. But I asked Nelimark about the possibility of undergoing at least some of the chemotherapy in Brookings as an outpatient. Nelimark consented and said that my treatment would begin at Brookings Hospital that night. Mom, Dad, and I then returned to Brookings and readied ourselves for what would begin later that night. In the meantime, I contacted Valerian, Chris, and others and made them aware of the situation. They helped me get in touch with university officials to withdraw from classes. I hated having my education interrupted again. But since there was no way of knowing how long I would remain in the hospital, it only made sense to withdraw from classes and receive a refund.

Nelimark was right; the treatment regimen was different from the previous ones. Rather than having two drugs administered continuously over seven days, I would receive only one chemotherapy drug, Ara-C. And the chemo wouldn't be infused every day; it would be delivered to me through the Hickman catheter every other day. Regardless of what the regimen was, I was happy that I would be able to stave off another potentially lengthy hospital stay for at least a few days more. My reprieve, however, would prove short-lived.

That evening, Mom and Dad took me to the hospital, and I went to a room where the chemotherapy would be administered. Total infusion time was going to be two to three hours. I liked the idea of having to be prostrate and having my mobility limited because of the chemotherapy infusion about as much as I liked the limitations imposed upon me during blood transfusions. At least I could lie down on a bed and watch TV.

I laid on the bed, and a nurse soon came to my bedside and prepared to give me some Benadryl intravenously. Once she gave me the injection via my Hickman catheter, she put the transparent bag of Ara-C on the IV pole and prepared to connect the bag to one of the ports of my catheter. I looked up at the bag and studied it, never having really paid much attention to IV bags before. On one side of the bag was a warning to medical personnel to wear latex gloves when handling chemotherapeutic drugs. In finer print, the warning cautioned that getting chemo drugs on hands could lead to skin irritation and a host of other maladies. I chuckled to myself. It's not OK for anyone to get chemo drugs on his or her skin. But it's perfectly all right for the stuff to be pumped directly into my heart and circulated throughout my body. Funny that.

I endured the first dose of chemotherapy with little trouble. I experienced the usual host of side effects, but they weren't altogether severe. In the following days, though, I found myself almost wilting—my strength and my sense of well-being seemed to slip away with each successive day. I felt really lousy, and there was seemingly no relief. Sleep wasn't the answer, because I couldn't sleep well. And riding to Sioux Falls in the family van every other day proved torturous. Though the van rode fairly smoothly, the undulations of the southbound lanes of Interstate 29 exacerbated my nausea, and I couldn't get comfortable even when lying down in the van's rear seats.

After two doses of chemotherapy in the early part of the week, I decided I couldn't handle driving back and forth to Sioux Falls anymore. In the infusion center at McKennan, I was taken to a private room where I laid down for a few minutes. Dad was with me, and Nelimark joined us shortly thereafter. I never would have uttered what I did at any point prior, but I felt that I had no choice: I implored Nelimark to admit me to the hospital for the remainder of my treatment. Even though my blood counts were still in a safe-enough range to permit me to remain outside the hospital, I had decided I would feel better being under the hospital's constant care. Nelimark consented, and I was once again admitted to the hospital. Dad followed me up to my new room in 3 East and helped me get settled in. He then contacted Mom and broke the news to her. She joined us at the hospital as soon as she got off work. Once again, none of us had any idea what the future had in store for me. But we were able to take comfort in knowing that the latest round of chemo was almost over. Only time would tell if it would put me into a durable remission.

13

Change of Course

While I was in the hospital, Mom and Dad visited me at least once a day. I had my share of other visitors as well. One regular "visitor," of course, was Nelimark. During one of his visits, Mom, Dad, the doctor, and I began discussing what lay in store for the remainder of my leukemia treatment. The key topic was a bone marrow transplant.

As soon as Mom, Dad, and I had returned from the Mayo Clinic in early October, Dad began doing research on bone marrow transplants. He contacted the National Marrow Donor Registry to see what information he could find. The registry sent him a guide to the various bone marrow transplant centers throughout the world. It described each center in detail, including the number of the various types of bone marrow transplants that each of the centers had performed.

When Nelimark talked about me undergoing a bone marrow transplant, he initially suggested the transplant be performed at the Mayo Clinic. Dad objected. According to Dad's research, the Mayo Clinic had performed only about one-tenth as many unrelated-donor transplants as the University of Minnesota. Nelimark protested, saying that numbers aren't really that important. He and Dad had a heated discussion about where the transplant would take place. I felt weary and implored Dad to stop arguing. But Dad stood his ground, and I'm glad he did. Nelimark relented, and we established that the transplant would take place at the University of Minnesota, assuming a suitable donor could be found.

Blood samples had already been drawn for locating a donor through the Mayo Clinic. Additional blood had to be drawn to prepare for a transplant at the University of Minnesota. Ideally, the resulting blood samples would generate a pool of probable candidates to be bone marrow donors for me.

Nelimark explained that in seeking out donors for bone marrow transplant patients, matching is done using six HLA antigens. Initial blood draws make it possible to match the first four of the six antigens. It's relatively easy to match the antigens and doing so can generate a pool of potential donors. From there, the potential donors are contacted to see if they are willing to consent to further testing to see if their remaining fifth and sixth antigens match the patient's. If the potential donors consent, they provide more blood samples, and the blood samples are tested to learn if the remaining two antigens match. If at least one of the candidates is a match, he or she is asked once again if he or she is willing to go through with the bone marrow donation. Assuming that the patient is in remission and is prepared for the transplant, a date is set, and marrow is withdrawn from the donor within twenty-four hours of the transplant.

Once I was admitted to the hospital after my relapse, I spent another month in McKennan. My experiences during this stay were much like those I had during previous admissions. I felt weaker than I ever had before and was content to spend most of my time lying in bed. I hated not being able to get out and be among people, but I didn't have enough gumption to get out of bed and do something. Nelimark encouraged me to get out of bed at least once a day and walk the halls. He said that if I didn't maintain some level of physical activity, I likely would need some kind of physical therapy during my stay in the hospital. I heeded his advice and made it a point to walk around the halls of 3 East at least once a day. I usually took my daily walks around the time

Mom and Dad came to visit. They visited nearly every day, only missing when winter weather wouldn't permit the hundred-mile round-trip.

Watching television and attempting to sleep occupied the next several days. A bone marrow biopsy performed within ten days after the conclusion of chemotherapy revealed that I was once again in remission. Nelimark, my parents, and I were again hopeful. The doctor said that I would be released from the hospital when my counts reached a safe level. To make sure my remission remained durable until the bone marrow transplant, he said I would need outpatient chemotherapy periodically. Nelimark assured us that the chemotherapy could be delivered in Brookings if we so chose.

During one of their evening visits to the hospital, my parents mentioned that Valerian or someone else at SDSU had asked me to prepare some kind of statement for the Native American Club. I was never told what the statement was for, but I later learned the reason behind the request. Likewise, I learned after the powwow why Valerian and others had been so insistent that I make it to the powwow, assuming that I was healthy enough.

In the few remaining days before the powwow, I was totally impotent to help. Chris and other club members who came to visit totally understood the situation. They picked up the slack that had resulted from my sickness and hospitalization. Chris and a few others had assumed my duties as secretary/treasurer, and everything was working out as planned. The only aspect of the powwow that caused concern for the club was that both Valerian and I would not be at the powwow. I was still hospitalized, and Valerian had to go to Ecuador for an International Partnership for Service-Learning annual conference, so he was out of the picture.

The morning Valerian left for Ecuador, he called me at the hospital from the airport around seven. His flight for South America would leave a few hours later. Calling me at that hour was all right because a nurse had awakened me a few hours earlier to draw blood and weigh me, and I had been unable to go back to sleep. In the meantime, I occupied myself with episodes of *Pokemon* on TV. When Valerian called, he told me he was preparing to leave, and he wanted to wish me well before he took off. It was good to hear from him, and I wished him a safe journey.

A few days later, the powwow came and went. Chris told me there were a few hiccups in the operation of the powwow, but there always are. Generally, everything worked out well: there were lots of drums and lots of dancers, and the club at least broke even on the event.

There was one surprise related to the powwow that I didn't learn about until my parents visited later that day. Mom and Dad reported than an honoring song had been sung for me, and that was why so many people had hoped I would be able to attend. I didn't get to experience the honoring firsthand, but Mom and Dad attended in my place. And my Lakota instructor videotaped the honoring for me, so I could watch it later. I was moved that the club members and others within the SDSU community regard me so highly as to have an honoring song for me. Later I learned that it was my friend Judy who asked one of the drum groups at the powwow to sing the honoring song. And with some help from my mom, Valerian and Chris compiled enough information about me that the Native American Club president, who emceed the powwow, could talk about my life and accomplishments before the honor song began.

More than a year after the powwow, I visited with Judy and thanked her for her gesture. Judy explained the motivation (along with friendship) behind her making an offering on my behalf. During one of her visits to the FacLab, I had worked with her on some projects for one of her classes. I had recently come home from the hospital, and we had talked that day about the hardships of the leukemia treatment and what may lie ahead for me. Judy said one thing I said about the arduousness of all the chemotherapy I had undergone really impressed her: "The only other choice is to die." I didn't realize my words would have such an effect on her or on others around me. Regardless, I was moved by Judy's honoring of me during the powwow.

Within a few weeks after the powwow, which occurred in the middle of February, my counts returned to a safe level, and I was able to return home from the hospital. I was happy to know that I was once again in remission. There was no way of knowing, however, whether the remission would be durable. I tried to return to as normal a life as possible, but huge questions loomed about if and when a donor for me would be found. There was nothing to do but wait.

14

A Surprising Phone Call

When I returned home from McKennan, my out-of-hospital routine changed little from what it had been after other hospital stays. I went back to work at the FacLab as I was able, and in general worked to make myself as useful as possible. I also attended Valerian's Introduction to American Indian Studies class. I had withdrawn from the university once again weeks before, so I didn't receive any credit for the work I did in the class. But going to class—especially one I enjoyed—gave me something on which to focus, other than the daily grind of my health.

It was midterm time at SDSU when I was released from the hospital in late February. Perhaps it was arrogance on my part, but I thought it would be fun to take Valerian's midterm and see how well I could do. Since I had gone through much of the material before and learned it from other sources (including Valerian, albeit in a different context), I was confident I would get a good grade. Being a good friend, Valerian indulged me in my request, and I took the midterm with the rest of the class. I got an A on the exam—not a high A, but an A nonetheless.

Midterms came and went, and work at the FacLab and in Valerian's class continued. I also continued my work for the Native American Club. The powwow, which is always the club's biggest event, was over, so there was little to which we needed to devote our collective efforts for the rest of the semester. But we still met at least once per month. During one of our meetings, the club discussed my health situation as a matter of business. Nicomas asked how much time I might have until I relapsed again. There was no good way to answer her question, but I speculated that it could be two months since two months had elapsed between the time when I finished my last round of chemotherapy and when I relapsed. My answer raised a great deal of concern among the club members. After the meeting, Nicomas, Chris, and others began working to rally people to get tested as potential donors for a transplant. I have no idea if anyone signed up, but the show of concern for me and people's desire to help was very touching.

In the weeks that followed, I continued to attend Valerian's class when I could. I made regular doctor visits to Sioux Falls and had blood and blood product transfusions as needed. I also continued to work at the FacLab as I was able. Of course, I did a lot of waiting in the meantime, waiting for a phone call telling me that a suitable donor had been found.

One surprising phone call came in March from the National Marrow Donor Registry. But the call wasn't to tell me that a donor for me had been found. The call came because I had provided a sample of blood during the SDSU powwow a few years earlier.

"Good morning, Mr. Whitehead," the woman on the other end of the line began, "I'm calling to let you know that you're a potential donor for someone awaiting a bone marrow transplant and would like to know if you're willing to consent to further testing."

Of course, I would have been more than willing to help someone in a similar situation if the circumstances were different. But given my state of affairs, helping out someone else was impossible.

"Well, I'd sure like to be able to help out like that," I said, sheepishly. "You're probably not going to believe this, but I'm actually waiting on a bone marrow donor myself."

There was silence for a moment, but she came back to the phone, and we talked about my health situation. We visited for a few minutes more, and she said she totally understood why I wouldn't be able to help. She also said that our visit was the first time she had ever contacted someone who needed a bone marrow donor himself or herself. She wished me luck with my search. I would receive another phone call from the National Marrow Donor Registry, but not for another month or so.

15

A Donor Is Found

Within a few weeks of the initial phone call from the National Marrow Donor Registry, I began undergoing outpatient chemotherapy. Nelimark said it would be all right if I received the chemo in Brookings. I was happy to hear such news and hoped that having more chemotherapy wouldn't require me to go back into the hospital. It didn't. I only had to have the outpatient chemotherapy a few times during the month, and I never really experienced any side effects. My black, spiky hair had begun to grow back, and the chemotherapy that I received seemed to leave the hair intact. There would be no need for me to have my head shaved because my hair was falling out until I got to Fairview University Medical Center in Minneapolis.

Each dose of Ara-C that I was given at the Brookings Hospital required about three to four hours to infuse. When I received the infusions, I would lay resting in the hospital's intensive care unit. I don't know why they infused me in intensive care; the only machine used was the infusion machine. The hospital staff likely put me in there because it was not in use by anyone else, and it was quiet and private. The unit was indeed quiet, and it was nice to be able to lie on a bed and sleep during the infusion. But the nicest aspect of the chemotherapy was knowing I could leave the hospital as soon as it was finished.

My day-to-day routine hadn't changed all that much since I had been released from 3 East at Avera McKennan in February. I worked when I could, attended Valerian's Introduction to American Indian

Studies course, and went to Native American Club meetings. Around the time I finished my outpatient chemotherapy, April had begun, and the spring semester had only a few weeks to go. The Native American Club was planning a fry bread and *wojapi* feed at the Wesleyan Church.

The Native American Club had been invited to prepare a meal for church members in exchange for some funds. The feed was going to be on a Friday afternoon, so most of the club prepared the fry bread the night before. It was good to feel strong enough and healthy enough to be out among people, and it felt good to be able to do something of service. We began around 6:00 PM and spent about four hours working on the fry bread and *wojapi*, a Lakota/Dakota/Nakota traditional fruit pudding often served with fry bread. Roughly half of our crew assembled the blueberries, sugar, and other ingredients needed to make the *wojapi*, and the rest of us devoted our time to making the bread dough and frying the bread.

We served the meal to more than a hundred Wesleyan Church members, and they hastily downed the food. Everyone seemed to enjoy it, and we made some extra money for the club. I was surprised that many church members seemed to know who I was and were aware of my condition. They were curious, and I tried to answer their questions as we all enjoyed the meal we had prepared. As we tidied things up for the evening, many people came to wish me well and assured me that they would pray for me.

I spent the next few days preparing for the American Indian studies final exam, which would be on a Tuesday night. It's not as though the outcome of the exam would have any impact on my grade-point average, since I wasn't receiving credit for the class. But I still wanted to perform as competently as I could. In the meantime, the Russell Crowe movie *Gladiator* had just come to town, and Valerian and I made plans to see it after we finished with the final exam that evening.

Tuesday afternoon came, and I studied for the exam after I got home from work at the FacLab. While I was working, an important phone call came. The person said that a suitable bone marrow donor had been found and suggested I get in touch with Nelimark to make plans for what would be a four-month stay in Minneapolis. She explained that I would have to remain in Minneapolis for one hundred days after the transplant. In spite of the good news, my heart sank. Having to live in Minneapolis—both in the hospital and in some other dwelling—would be difficult. I would be away from most of my friends and family. Still, I knew the stay was necessary, especially considering that the bone marrow transplant likely was key to my long-term survival of leukemia. After answering a few other questions, the caller told me I would need to visit the University of Minnesota a few times in the following weeks so that my overseeing physician could examine me and determine what treatment regimen would be required. My first visit to the Twin Cities would be in two weeks. The caller and I exchanged good-byes, and I set out to tell Dad, Mom, and others the good news.

I was certainly excited when I arrived early for class that night. I always like to arrive early for happenings anyway, but I wanted to make sure I would have enough time to tell Valerian about the new development in my life. Valerian was happy to hear the news. I finished the exam in a little over an hour. I was among the last to finish because I always check my work. I turned in my exam, Valerian filed it away with the other test papers, and we headed for the movie theater.

Before *Gladiator* began, Valerian and I discussed how I thought the exam went and the events of the past few days. I was excited that the semester was over, and Valerian seemed to be as well. The greatest excitement for me, however, was knowing that a bone marrow donor had been found. I did feel some sense of dread at having to be away from everyone in Brookings and the surrounding communities for a

period of time. But I still didn't have any fear of death; I was more concerned about what life during the transplant experience would be like,
as well as about how life after the transplant would be affected. The
future was a question.

After the movie, Valerian and I parted for the evening. I was tired
from all of the events and excitement of the day. But I felt good going
to sleep that night, knowing that I had just taken a tremendous step
forward in beating cancer. Whether everything would work out
remained to be seen.

A sunny April day a few weeks later, Mom, Dad, and I made our way
to the Twin Cities. Those at the hospital with whom we had spoken
said the required testing would take a few days. We found a hotel close
to the hospital and got down to business.

The battery of tests that I underwent over the next few days was quite
rigorous. Fortunately, I had a good deal of strength and stamina, so the
tests weren't too difficult. In addition to the obvious blood tests and bone
marrow biopsy, I had a lung function test and an MRI. I never really
knew the purpose of such tests and can only assume that the results would
help the doctors and nurses predict how well I would withstand the bone
marrow transplant. The numbers also probably provided a baseline for
how my body functioned prior to the transplant.

None of the tests was difficult to endure, but the bone marrow
biopsy was somewhat painful. It was less painful than the other biopsies
I'd had but still hurt somewhat. The key difference was that I was anes-
thetized before the University of Minnesota physicians performed the
biopsy, and in Sioux Falls, I had been treated only with local anesthet-
ics. At the University of Minnesota, I received up to 50 mg of Demerol
intravenously and a local anesthetic at the biopsy site.

When the doctors in the Phillips-Wangensteen building gave me the
Demerol, it put me into a state of being doped-up that I had never

experienced. With previous lower doses of Demerol and morphine, I had felt like I was flying, but I had never felt such chemically induced euphoria until 50 mg of the narcotic was administered. I became sleepy and could easily have passed off into sleep if the doctors and nurses hadn't continued talking to me. As the sleepiness lessened, warm feelings of comfort and punchiness overwhelmed me. Rather than making me quiet and complacent, the Demerol seemed to loosen my tongue and make me more talkative. I've never been drunk, but I imagine that what I experienced under such a high dose of narcotics is similar to what I would experience if I were to get drunk. It's strange, though, that I'm able to remember events that happened under the influence of the anesthetic.

I recall that one of the other doctors who performed the biopsy didn't have enough physical strength to penetrate the bone. It wasn't in my medical records, but the doctors became aware that I have a very hard skeleton when the first doctor who attempted to do the biopsy couldn't finish the job. I lay on a table that was roughly at waist level with the young doctor. She leaned over me, made a small incision in my lower back, and began trying to puncture my bone with the aspirating needle. She tried several times but was unable to muster the strength needed. I felt kind of bad for that doctor; I hope she wasn't penalized for not being able to do the biopsy.

Another doctor came in to finish the job. He performed the biopsy with little trouble, and I was soon allowed to remain in the room to sleep off the lingering effects of the Demerol. Mom and Dad stayed in the room with me for a while and then retired to the waiting room as I lay on an examination table under dim incandescent lights. It took about half an hour for me to get back to normal and be released from the clinic. We were told that a bone marrow transplant coordinator would contact me within a few days. Mom, Dad, and I took an elevator to the hospital cafeteria. We had a quick bite to eat, loped back to our car, and made our way back to Brookings. It was the middle of spring, so it was starting to get dark by the time we got home. But there was still more light than there had been many times before when I returned home from Avera McKennan.

When I prepared to rest for the night, I knew that the transplant was drawing near. There was likely still at least a month before the transplant, but the time was coming ever closer. I hoped I had enough time to prepare for the four-month-long venture that would soon follow. Fortunately, Mom and Dad were handling the practical and financial preparations for the transplant. My own preparations involved spending as much time as possible with close friends and family and preparing myself psychologically and spiritually for the next leg of my leukemia journey. It's hard to prepare when one doesn't know what's ahead, but I did the best I could.

16

Tests, Tests, and More Tests

A few days after I returned from my first visit to the University of Minnesota, I had made plans to have coffee with Velva-Lu. We agreed that we would meet in the student union on Tuesday morning before I went to work in the FacLab and catch up on what had been happening in each other's lives.

Tuesday morning came, and I began my routine as I had so many times before. I slipped out of bed and into some clothes, flushed the two ports of my Hickman catheter with saline, and had a bowl of cereal as I watched a rerun of *Knight Rider* on the USA Network. Everything seemed to go according to plan.

Shivering in the chill of the bathroom, I disrobed and stepped into the shower. I put a few dabs of shampoo into my left hand and began to work it into my scalp and what little hair I had. Eyes closed, I massaged my scalp a bit and adjusted the flow of warm water. It was then that I heard something unusual.

Clink!

I thought something had fallen off one of the ledges in the shower. When I looked down, I saw my Hickman catheter on the floor of the bathtub at my feet. My eyes then went to the clear plastic patch that covered the part of my chest where the catheter had once dangled. There was a little blood seeping out of the hole the tubing had occupied. On one level, I felt relieved to not have the blasted thing protruding from my chest. But I was afraid of the possibility of infection. I felt a sense of urgency as I showered as quickly as I could and dried off so I could get to the phone. First, I called Velva-Lu to let her know that I probably wouldn't make it for coffee that day. She wasn't in the office, so I left a message.

My next call was to Nelimark. My fear of infection had been replaced with good feelings for being relieved of the catheter. At the same time, I wanted to see if Nelimark would want to install another catheter. I got in touch with him right away, and he said installing another catheter wasn't necessary.

"They'll put another one in in Minneapolis anyway," Nelimark assured me.

It took me a few minutes to calm down after losing the catheter and talking with my doctor. But once I did, I got dressed and ready for work. At work I was finally able to get in touch with Velva-Lu, who was very concerned about me.

The following days passed quickly. I worked with quite a few faculty members in the FacLab, and everyone who passed through was happy to see that I was in good spirits and good health, even if only for the time being. It buoyed my spirits to have so many people interested in my well-being and showing their support.

A few weeks later, Dad and I returned to Minneapolis to meet with doctors and with the bone marrow transplant coordinator to learn more of the specifics of what my treatment regimen would be. Mom had to stay home and work. And it was OK that Mom didn't go with us; there wasn't anything we learned that we couldn't recount to her later.

Dad and I first met with Dr. Philip McGlave, who would act as my overseeing physician. He explained that when the time came for me to be prepared for the transplant, I would undergo two days of chemo-therapeutic treatment using the drug cyclophosphamide, also known as Cytoxan. Once the chemo was over, I would receive fifteen minutes of full-body irradiation twice a day for four days. I would then have a day of rest before the transplant. He explained that I would remain in the hospital until my neutrophil count reached a safe level. After my release from the hospital, I would remain in the Minneapolis area for whatever the remainder of one hundred days would be. That's assuming, of course, that I wasn't readmitted to the hospital or didn't survive. McGlave also said that my preparations would begin May 24, which was only a few weeks away. During my admission to the hospital, another Hickman catheter would be installed.

After meeting with McGlave, Dad and I went to a conference room and met with a bone marrow transplant coordinator. There were three or four other sets of people in this meeting, many of whom were parents with young children. The coordinator explained some of the costs involved with the transplant process, as well as what people could expect in going through the transplant. Before we left, he gave each of us a thick, three-ring binder containing past editions of a national bone marrow transplant newsletter. I think we were meant to assume that the information contained in the binders would cover all the bases with regards to what might happen with bone marrow transplants. In retrospect, there was a lot I experienced and underwent that the information didn't cover. It may be impossible to cover all bases, but it would have been nice to have a lot of the blanks filled in.

Dad and I again visited the hospital cafeteria and had a quick bite to eat before we headed back to Brookings. Both of us were kind of keyed up from receiving so much crucial information, but we regained our composures enough to enjoy a decent meal before we hit the road. Of all the information we received, the most pertinent at that time was when the process would begin. That date was fast approaching. We had our work cut out for us, and we knew exactly how much time we had to prepare.

17

Heading into the Unknown

In the weeks that followed, my routine was much the same as it had been for the previous months. The key difference was, now that classes were done, I no longer needed to be concerned about schoolwork. It would have been nice to attend summer classes if I were in good health. But summer classes—or classes of any kind—would have to wait.

When I had the energy and the drive to do so, I pored through the three-ring binder of materials that I had received at the University of Minnesota. The information largely pertained to side effects that I could expect as a result of the bone marrow transplant and about complications such as graft-versus-host disease. There were also pamphlets and flyers about support groups for patients and caregivers.

One point that the bone marrow transplant coordinator emphasized during our Minnesota meeting was that once I was released from the hospital, there was no way I would be in any condition to support and take care of myself. I would need a caregiver. We decided that Dad would live with me in Minneapolis and act as my caregiver. Mom wanted to be there with us, too, but we decided it would be best if she remained in South Dakota and come to Minnesota when she was able.

Mom, through her employment at Sioux Valley Energy, was our principal wage earner and was the one working to keep our health insurance in effect. Things were difficult financially because of my leukemia, but it would have been much worse without insurance. The transplant alone cost in excess of $150,000. And the total cost of all of my treatments over a year-and-a-half period exceeded $1.25 million.

There was so much material to wade through, but I really didn't spend all that much time reading the newsletters in the three-ring binder. If nothing else, the stories about people who had gone through and survived bone marrow transplants provided me with additional hope that I would survive, too. Looking back, I believe that the information in the binder only scratched the surface regarding what to expect from the bone marrow transplant process.

A few weeks later, with Mom's assistance, Dad and I loaded the car and made yet another journey toward the Twin Cities. This time I would not return to South Dakota for several weeks. Rather than head directly to the hospital, we stopped at the home of my uncle Gene, who lives in Cottage Grove, Minnesota. We planned to spend the night at his house, before I entered the hospital the next day.

Dad, Uncle Gene, and I spent what remained of the day hanging out at the house, trying to prepare ourselves for what lay ahead. We had no idea what the outcome would be, but we did the best we could to humor each other and keep our thoughts positive. We missed Mom, but we took comfort in knowing that she would join us in a few days. Meanwhile, I popped in the videotape of my honoring at the powwow. Gene and Dad seemed to enjoy watching the video, but I felt a bit embarrassed by all the attention. Still, I was glad I had included the powwow tape among various drumming videos that I had brought with me to amuse myself during what would likely be a long stay in the hospital. If nothing else, the honoring video would remind me of how many people were supporting me in what I was about to undergo.

I knew I likely wouldn't get to drive again for some time, so I took the van out for a cruise as darkness began to settle over the eastern suburbs of the Twin Cities. Because I didn't know the area well, I stayed near the neighborhoods of Cottage Grove. As I drove, I listened to songs from CDs I had picked up recently. Among the selections were "Relax" by Frankie Goes to Hollywood and "Stand Beside Me" by Kansas. Driving the van in unfamiliar territory wasn't as fun as, say, running my Nissan NX2000 through a racecourse, but my options were limited. I enjoy driving, and I knew it would likely be weeks, if not months, before I could slip behind the wheel of a fun car again.

When I returned to Gene's place that night after I had picked up what would be my last order of McDonald's french fries for a while, Dad and Gene were watching TV. It was getting late, but not so late that the evening news shows were on. We all sat and relaxed as best we could. In the meantime, I thumbed through the materials the hospital had given me. As I put everything aside and readied myself for bed, I thought, *I'm ready for this*. Over the following several weeks, I learned that I could never have been more wrong.

18

Countdown to Day Zero

The following morning, Uncle Gene, Dad, and I braved rush-hour traffic on I-94 West and made our way toward the University of Minnesota campus. Traffic was heavy, but not insurmountably so. Door-to-door, the journey took less than half an hour. We arrived at the hospital on time, and I was admitted in relatively short order.

I was taken to a large, open room. Curtains cordoned off the examining tables, but there was little privacy. One of the nurses took me to one of the cordoned areas, and I was given a gown to change into. Meanwhile, Dad remained in the waiting area. I discreetly slipped out of my sweatpants and T-shirt and into the gown as I waited for someone to install an IV in my arm. I wouldn't need the IV for long, but I would need it for the procedure during which a new Hickman catheter would be installed in my chest.

Before long, a nurse installed the IV. And then the waiting began. It felt like an eternity before a doctor finally came with a gurney to take me to the room where the catheter would be installed. It was really only a half hour, but given my apprehension and anxiety, it felt like an eternity. The doctor gave me an injection of morphine through the IV. He also explained that I would undergo an additional procedure before being taken to my hospital room. He told me that about a liter of my own bone marrow would be aspirated. There were two reasons for removing some of my original marrow: one was for research purposes because the University of Minnesota hospital is a research hospital. The second reason was in case the new bone marrow failed to engraft, my original marrow could be reinfused to keep me alive long enough to find another suitable donor.

The next thing I knew, I was lying in a hospital bed on the fourth floor of the Fairview University Medical Center. Dad sat at my side, and a new Hickman catheter protruded from the right side of my chest. I had hoped they'd put the catheter in the left side of my chest so that I would have matching scars on both sides of my chest, but no such luck.

Dad and I visited for a while, and then a doctor joined us to discuss what would happen over the next several days. The plan was for me to undergo two days of chemotherapy and then four days of full-body irradiation. The chemo and the radiation would wipe out what was left of my original bone marrow and prepare the linings of my long bones to receive the new marrow.

Chemotherapy was nothing new to me, but the cautions required in the administration of Cytoxan were new. Cytoxan is so toxic, the doctor told me, that I would need to urinate every two hours. The chemo is metabolized quickly and then excreted from the body through urination. However, it is so toxic that it could eat away at the lining of my bladder if it were allowed to sit there for very long. The doctor said the chemotherapy would begin the following day.

He then explained what the full-body irradiation would be like. It really didn't sound all that bad, but there was always the possibility of side effects. Some of the side effects, such as weakness and nausea, were more immediate. Others, such as an increased likelihood of developing other forms of cancer or cataracts, were more long-term.

Not long after he finished talking about the radiation, the doctor left. By that time, the sun was beginning to lower itself in the sky. Dad sat with me for a little while longer and then retired for the night. I was alone. Dad would return for a while the next day, but I would then be left alone for a few days as Dad went back to Brookings to collect some needed items and return with Mom.

I tried to relax that night but was unable to do so. I don't understand why I had so much difficulty sleeping; it wasn't as though I felt particularly anxious. But the bed was uncomfortable, and I was confined—albeit for my own protection—in an isolated and uncomfortable environment. I tossed and turned throughout the night and found myself often glancing at the soft green glow of the VCR's digital clock.

A few times throughout the night, I called for the nurse and asked if she could give me some medication to help me sleep. The nurse left and returned with a few milligrams of Ativan. Unfortunately, the drug didn't seem to work; sleep eluded me for most of the night. As the night wore on, I began to develop severe pains in my lower back. They gave me hot packs, which helped some, but I remained in pain. Not getting much sleep that night was a bad way to begin the bone marrow transplant process.

The following morning, I did my best to seem awake and lively. But in reality, I had a lot of trouble appearing vigorous. No one could blame me, really. A nurse brought me my breakfast, and I ate what little I could. There was nothing wrong with the food, but I didn't have much appetite.

A short time later, another nurse came to me and told me to get out of bed and take a shower. I wasn't in the mood to shower, but the nurse was insistent; I really didn't have a choice in the matter. So into the shower I went. When the shower was done, she broke out the electric razor and shaved me bald, at my request. I knew my hair was going to fall out anyway, so I figured it would be better to cut it off. While the nurse cut my hair, her demeanor seemed to soften. She was gentle in cutting my hair. The nurse then left me alone as I waited for the chemotherapy.

Before the end of the morning, a nurse came in with an IV bag full of Cytoxan and connected it to the IV pole from which several other bags and apparatuses hung. In addition to the traditional saline IV, there was a bag of TPN (total parenteral nutrition) that would nourish me during my stay in the hospital. There was also a morphine pump that I could trigger if I experienced severe pain. There were times when I was in a good deal of pain, but the morphine seemed to do little good. I know the amount of morphine I could have in a given period of time was controlled, but still, the amount of morphine on which I could draw was supposed to be enough to quell pain. In every instance I used the pump, I found the pain relief inadequate.

It took a while before I began to notice any nausea or other side effects from the chemotherapy. But as the day went on, I began to experience stomach sickness. And almost like clockwork, every two hours, a nurse would enter the room and help me to the bathroom to empty my bladder. The time of day or night made no difference. My regular visits to the bathroom continued around the clock until after the chemotherapy was finished. Other than the pain in my lower back, I didn't feel much pain.

The following day, after I had awakened and emptied the contents of my stomach, I mustered the strength to look out the window and survey the hospital's surroundings. When I was admitted, one of the nurses had told me I would be able to see a great view of the Mississippi River. I couldn't see the river at all.

As the day wore on, I became agitated about being forced to remain confined to the room. The feeling was much like what I had experienced at Avera McKennan. Only this time, the feeling was more intense and was coupled with fear and loneliness. I understood why Mom and Dad wouldn't be up to visit me right away; they needed to get a few things ready before they could come to the hospital and join me. But during that time, my longing for my parents, friends, and anything remotely familiar grew stronger.

In the afternoon, I made many futile attempts to sleep, not so much because I was tired, but I wanted to drift off into a state where all that was happening to me would seem far away, even if only for a few hours. I had no luck in sleeping, though, so I entertained myself by flipping through myriad TV stations. I couldn't find anything I wanted to watch, so I popped in a few videotapes. The first was *Liquid Drum Theater*, which was Mike Portnoy's two-tape instructional video, during which he talked about the recording of the songs of Liquid Tension Experiment and some recent Dream Theater albums. The other tape was *Star Wars Episode I: The Phantom Menace.*

In the midst of *Episode I*, Uncle Gene popped in to see how I was doing. It was good to see a familiar face, and I enjoyed his company. While we visited, Uncle Gene asked if there was anything he could do or get for me. I had not yet lost my sense of taste, so I craved something other than bland hospital fare. And comfort food certainly was in order, so I asked if he could get me a grilled cheese sandwich from the hospital cafeteria. Uncle Gene was happy to comply, and I downed the sandwich as we visited.

Daylight soon gave way to evening, and I was faced with the prospect of another sleepless night. I took some comfort that I wasn't exceedingly nauseated by the chemotherapy that was flowing through my circulatory system. It was cold comfort, though. I was still frightened deep down inside about facing a situation with an unknowable outcome and about being physically separated from so many people who had supported me while I was in Sioux Falls. When I was in Avera McKennan, most of my friends were only about an hour's drive away and could visit me fairly easily. In Minneapolis, a four-hour drive across western Minnesota separated me from many of the people about whom

I cared. I knew a few friends in the Minneapolis area, but I only saw one, my old friend Ben. I e-mailed a few others about being in Minneapolis, but they replied that they wouldn't visit me because they "don't go to hospitals."

Before attempting to sleep, I tried to soothe myself by writing on the Toshiba laptop computer that Mom and Dad had given me the year before. I had used the laptop to write most of my papers and do most of my Internet surfing while I was in the journalism program. I also used the laptop to do a fair bit of Web design work for ITC.

I didn't have a lot of physical stamina, so I didn't do much writing. And I had only a dial-up Internet connection from my hospital room, so I easily lost patience in trying to connect with others via e-mail. I wrote what little I could and tried to be as complete as I could in what I wrote. As I wrote, I entertained myself with some of my CDs. One that I remember playing was the second disc of Rush's *Chronicles*. One track on the disc that I had come to love was "Subdivisions." Most of the enjoyment I derived from the song stemmed from hearing Neil Peart's drumming. But the dark, menacing sounds of the analog synthesizers featured in the song, which came out in 1982, brought back memories of my childhood. I didn't start listening to Rush in earnest until I was in my late teens, and I don't recall hearing "Subdivisions" when I was a kid. The connection to my childhood, I believe, was that the synthesizer sound reminded me of the sound tracks of the multitude of video arcade games I played in my youth. Regardless of what the connection was, the song had an effect on me that night in the hospital that it never had had before—it made me weep. I think the song caused me to cry because it offered me at least some small connection to my life back home, to the world I knew. It was one thin thread connecting me to my home and the life I had left behind.

Another lonely and sleepless night passed. This time, however, the source of my sleeplessness wasn't anxiety; it was lower back pain. The hot packs the nurses offered me provided some relief but not much. My morphine pump didn't really help, either. My hospital bed mattress felt uncomfortable, so I decided to try the cot, which had been brought in so my parents could stay with me in the hospital room when they returned. The cot sat in a dark corner of the room. My back didn't feel quite as sore when I moved to the cot, but it wasn't much of an improvement. At least it offered a different vantage point from which to stare at the ceiling.

In time, I must have fallen asleep briefly. When I came to, I felt very confused. My mind conjured the thought that I was in an apartment building in Aurora, South Dakota. I don't know where such a thought came from, but that's where I thought I was. I don't really remember much about that night, apart from once staring out from the darkness and into the yellow light that filtered through the door's window and into the room. In that light, I saw the silhouette of a woman at the door. It likely was a nurse, but I don't know for sure.

The chemotherapy bag on my IV pole was disconnected not long after I awoke the next morning. The two days' worth of Cytoxan would turn out to be the last chemotherapy I would have, but my experience with full-body irradiation was only beginning.

Within a few hours of finishing the chemo, I was helped into a wheelchair and taken to a different area of the hospital. There I was helped onto a table and told to sit in a curled-up position in which my knees touched my chest. My arms and legs were bound so I could remain in that position. After I was properly positioned, one of the radiology technicians explained that each dose of radiation would take about fifteen minutes, and I would receive the doses twice a day. He told me that the only way I would be able to tell I was being irradiated would be a consistent buzzing noise that I would hear from one side of the room. And there definitely was buzzing. When the radiation dose was finished, I was put back into a wheelchair and returned to my room. I didn't feel any different after the radiation than I had felt before. But I had to remember that I had received only one dose. Side effects likely would come later.

One thing that kept my spirits high was knowing that my parents would be returning to stay with me through the transplant. The plan was that they would return to the Twin Cities by 5:00 PM. My next scheduled dose of radiation was slated for 4:00 PM. If I had to go through my first day of radiation alone, that was all right. The important thing was that Mom and Dad would be by my side before too long.

I was halfway through a *Simpsons* episode and was downing a tasteless portion of salad when Mom and Dad appeared at my doorway and came toward me with open arms. My fears of being in protective isolation disappeared, even if only for a while, but I once again began to cry. I hadn't expected to cry, but tears began streaming down my face. I had missed my parents so much and was so scared of my situation without them being there to support me. I had never cried when they visited me at Avera McKennan. But I cried when they arrived back in Minneapolis. My parents were a crucial connection to the familiar, to the life I had known back in South Dakota. Mom and Dad spent the night with me. They spent the remaining nights at Uncle Gene's house, except the night the transplant took place. Even if they weren't with me twenty-four hours a day, I took comfort in knowing that my parents were in the area. That was good enough for me.

The following day, I received another two doses of full-body irradiation. By the end of the day, my radiation treatments were half over.

And I was fewer than four days away from day zero, the day of the transplant itself.

I hadn't experienced any side effects from the radiation until the afternoon of the second day of treatments. That afternoon, as I lay in bed and tried to relax, I saw stars before my eyes and flashes of bright light like I had never seen before. My first thought was that it was a side effect of the radiation. I have no explanation for what caused me to see such things. That afternoon, an eye doctor visited me, examined me, and found nothing abnormal. The stars and flashes of light never recurred.

That night, I lay in bed for hours on end, as I had so many nights before, both in Fairview and in Avera McKennan. One would think that I would have been used to the insomnia, the tossing and turning, by then. But no such luck. I lay awake and looked at the digital clock on the VCR in the room; it read 1:34. I flipped on the TV for a few minutes and listened to the final few scenes of some British animated movie about a giant robot.

19

A Fall in the Night

In spite of all that had been done to my body, I didn't feel all that bad. I began losing my sense of taste (something that I didn't fully realize until I left the hospital and tried to eat some "real food"), and I felt very weak. But I didn't have mouth sores, and I didn't feel all that nauseated.

Mom and Dad spent a good chunk of the day with me and did their best to keep my mind focused on good things that were happening in life. They did what they could to remain cheerful, but inside, I'm sure they were experiencing their own personal hells. As the patient, I at least had some control over my treatment and how I handled all that I was experiencing. I was an active participant in fighting my illness. My parents, and everyone else, could do little apart from pray for me and support me in other ways. They didn't have a direct method of fighting this sickness with me, and that could certainly give rise to feelings of helplessness. I'm sure Mom and Dad weren't doing well emotionally at times, but they did their best to hide their inner turmoil. I'm sure they did so to protect me.

In the late hours of the day, probably around 11:30 that night, I found myself tossing and turning in bed. TV wasn't relaxing me so that I would go to sleep, so I called the nurse and asked if she could give me something to help me sleep. She entered the room, patiently listened to my complaint, and said she would give me a dose of Ativan. Ativan had never really worked for me, but I thought it couldn't hurt. I knew morphine would have effectively put me to sleep, but no morphine was available, apart from that doled out by my pump. So that option was out.

Before the nurse gave me the Ativan, I asked if she would help me to the restroom. It's not that I didn't have the strength to make it to the bathroom, which was no more than fifteen feet from my bed. But the distance was difficult to traverse because of my IV pole. The nurse disconnected the pole from the wall, helped me to my feet, and loped slowly ahead of me as we made our way toward the bathroom. The nurse reached the bathroom before I did and began trying to hasten the pole into the bathroom. She must not have noticed the thick brown rubber lip in the doorway between the room and the bathroom.

One of the four wheels of the IV pole hit the rubber lip, and the pole began to tip sideways. The pole and all of the bags and other apparatuses attached to it crashed to the floor. And since the IV pole had me on a short leash, I went down with the pole and landed on top of it, mainly hitting my chest and belly. I developed a nice Rorschach-test bruise on my belly. That bruise remained visible for more than a year.

"Oh my God!" the nurse exclaimed, as she scrambled to assess the damage to both the IV pole and my body. In the meantime, I still lay on top of the IV pole, groaning in pain. Fortunately, the fall looked worse than it was. I hadn't broken anything, but I was still in pain. No matter how many times I hit the button for my morphine pump, the pain wouldn't subside.

The nurse helped me to my feet and stood the IV pole back on its wheels. She apologized profusely as I made my way to the toilet and relieved myself. When I finished, the nurse helped me to my bed once again, apologizing the whole way. I told her I was all right and not to worry about what had happened. She helped me get comfortable, and within about twenty minutes, my pain went away. The nurse gave me some Ativan to help me sleep. But no matter how much I tried to relax, I couldn't go to sleep. The drug just wouldn't work for me.

As I had so many times before, I peered out of the darkness and looked ahead to check the time shown on the VCR's digital clock. The stiff, green numbers showed 2:16. *Oh, great,* I thought. After looking at the clock, I glanced out one of the windows in my room. The words spoken by one of my nurses continued to resonate in my skull: "You'll have a great view of the Mississippi River."

Yeah, right, I thought, as I turned away from the window once again. I could see little in the darkness, apart from the off-white fluorescent glow spilling in through the narrow window to my room.

20

"The Beginning of a Whole New Life"

Part of my treatment regimen was to have a day of rest between my last day of full-body irradiation and the bone marrow transplant. Early in the morning, nurses came in, checked my vital signs, and drew blood. Later in the day, a doctor visited with me and told me that the chemotherapy and radiation appeared to be working; my blood counts, particularly my white cell counts, were dwindling to nothing. It appeared that my bones were well on their way to being ready to accept the new marrow that would be infused early the next day. Whether the infused marrow would work was not known, but at least my body was responding well to treatment.

Mom and Dad spent much of the day with me. It was good to visit with them, and it made me feel better to have them at my side. There wasn't much that Mom or Dad or anyone else could do for me, but it was good to have company. As they had so many times before, Mom and Dad kept my spirits high and encouraged me and told me that everything would be all right. I didn't feel too frightened at that point, but I very badly wanted my parents to be right.

The day was clear and sunny, and I imagined that it was quite hot. I had been in the hospital almost a week, and I missed being able to be outside among other people and to feel the warmth of the sun on my face and body. *Those days will come again soon*, I told myself.

Morning gave way to afternoon. Both Mom and Dad had some errands to run, so they left me for a while. I entertained myself as best I could with sending and receiving e-mails and watching videos. It was hard to relax, but at least the videos provided some distraction.

The sun was still well above the horizon but was starting to sink as the day's *Simpsons* episode came on the tube. My supper arrived, but I already had started to lose my sense of taste, so the hospital fare was even less palatable than before. The ranch dressing on my salad was about the only thing that gave me pleasure.

That night was when the bone marrow transplant would take place. No one ever specified exactly when the transplant would take place, but I was told that it would happen sometime in the middle of the night. Ordinarily, neither my parents nor I would have been pleased about staying up so late to do something. In this case, we were more than happy to make an exception.

As I lay in my hospital bed visiting with my parents, I imagined what my donor, whoever she was, was doing at the time. I imagine that she was entering a hospital, being sedated, and getting ready to donate her marrow. Once the marrow was collected, it would be hand-delivered to the hospital. I had learned this from reading the literature the hospital had provided.

I felt pretty fatigued by the time 1:00 AM rolled around. We were sleepy, but all of us were filled with anticipation. We still didn't know for certain when the transplant would take place, but we understood that it would be soon. In the darkness of the hospital room, I tried to snooze, but to no avail. I visited with Mom and Dad for as long as I could, and the three of us did all we could to maintain our composure. I wasn't thinking about it at the time, but in hindsight, that night was one of the most important in my life.

Around half past one, a nurse came in with a bag of greenish-brown fluid and prepared to attach it to the IV pole. After the fluid was attached to the pole, the nurse visited with my parents and me for a few minutes before hooking the bag to my Hickman catheter.

"This will be the beginning of a whole new life for you," the nurse said, smiling. She asked my parents to huddle around me, and she shot a Polaroid picture of us. I don't imagine that the picture turned out very well, considering how dark it was in the room. But the composition of the photo probably wasn't important; the doctors and nurses likely wanted little more than a record of the occasion. I'm sure that they, like my parents and me, hoped that I would be one of the hospital's success stories. I don't know how many patients had preceded me in receiving such a procedure, but I later learned that the University of Minnesota had performed bone marrow transplants since 1968. In fact, I discovered while doing research for a class a few years later that the first bone marrow transplant ever was performed at the University of Minnesota.

I don't recall any sensations as the new marrow was infused into me. In fact, I don't remember much about the night after the Polaroid picture was taken. A sedative was administered before my infusion, and I must have fallen asleep during the procedure. Bone marrow has the consistency of thick blood, so I imagine it took about three or four hours to infuse the new marrow into my body. It's kind of funny, now that I think about it. I slept through what was likely one of the most important events of my life. I don't know if Mom and Dad remained awake, but I was out like a light.

Our chief concern from that point was whether the marrow would work. We had done all we could, and the outcomes were out of our hands. All we could do was hope.

21

The Start of One Hundred Days

I didn't feel any different the morning after the bone marrow transplant. As with the numerous bone marrow biopsies I had undergone under sedation, the procedure was over before I knew it began. All that remained was to hope that the new marrow would work and that my world would soon return to some semblance of normalcy.

Mom and Dad spent the morning with me and then left to run errands and rest. I watched television and videos. I felt pretty tired that morning and wanted to sleep, but knew that trying to nap would be fruitless. At least I could take comfort in the fact that the main event—the bone marrow transplant—had already occurred. And all would hopefully be well from there.

The following several days were surprisingly similar to one another. Day in and day out, I remained in my room and tried to recover from the bone marrow transplant. Despite feeling totally wiped out and weak, my desire to be active and to leave the hospital remained as strong as ever. Fortunately, the blood draws each day showed that the marrow was beginning to engraft, as indicated by my gradually increasing white blood cell count.

One key change was that more and more medicines were added to my regimen. Among the main ones were cyclosporine and 140 mg doses of prednisone. Both were intended to retard the growth of the bone marrow that was beginning to engraft. It's kind of a paradox: the desired result of the transplant would be for the bone marrow to start growing a new immune system inside my own body, but it would be bad if the growth occurred unchecked.

Both drugs seemed to accomplish their aims, but they also brought side effects that I hadn't known about until I started experiencing them. The cyclosporine made my hands tremble so badly that I had difficulty eating, drinking, and writing. The prednisone caused pronounced anxiety and a puffy face. Fortunately, all of these effects would dissipate as I tapered off the drugs over several months.

In the days after the bone marrow transplant, a nurse came in at least once a day and checked my blood sugar level. At the time, I didn't think to ask the nurses why my blood sugars were being checked. I knew diabetics were supposed to check their blood sugar levels, but it never occurred to me that I might be diabetic. I didn't realize that the prednisone raised my blood sugar to where I would require insulin shots. The nurse who helped me start the discharge process told me that I would see an endocrinologist. When I inquired why, she told me I was diabetic. Undergoing a bone marrow transplant wasn't enough. If I survived, I would have to live with diabetes. Fortunately, I learned about a year later that the diabetes was temporary; my blood sugars have been well within the normal range since I got off the prednisone in the spring of 2001.

I was hospitalized seventeen days after the transplant, but it didn't seem all that long. Still, I had been in the hospital about a month by that point and was eager to leave. I knew I needed to remain near the hospital for nearly three months more. The prospect of being away from home for so long certainly didn't appeal to me, but at least I would have some semblance of freedom and wouldn't be confined to protective isolation.

I was filled with anxiety and excitement the day I was to be released from Fairview. The excitement stemmed from knowing I was finally going back outside into the world again. Anxiety came from the high doses of prednisone I was taking.

In the later morning of that mid-June day, I sat in a corner waiting room with Mom and Dad as we waited for the nurses to gather my medications and instruct me on how to take them each day. It seemed like we waited forever, but it was probably no more than an hour. Mom and Dad seemed as happy as I was to leave the hospital, but I'm sure that both were nervous about what lay ahead. Social workers serving the hospital had arranged for Dad and me to move into a furnished apartment nearby. The future was uncertain, but we at least had a place to live.

A nurse finally came with my meds and explained what pills I needed to take. I would need to take about fifty pills a day until I was further notified. Luckily, many of the pills were small and could be easily swallowed with fluid. But some of the pills, like the cyclosporine capsules, were large and difficult to swallow.

Mom and Dad helped me into our car, and we headed toward our apartment. I had never lived in an apartment, so I didn't know what to expect. All that really mattered, though, was that we had a place to live, a place to serve as a base of operations as we remained in the Twin Cities for the next three months. Our apartment was on Franklin Avenue near downtown Minneapolis.

Before we pulled into the parking lot of the Cities 94 apartment complex, I asked Mom and Dad if I could have some "real food" before we settled in. At that time, "real food" meant a cheeseburger, fries, and a Coke from a nearby Wendy's. Mom and Dad were happy to comply but cautioned me to keep my mask on. I'm sure that I drew a lot of attention when I stepped into the restaurant, especially since I was also sickly white and hairless. But I didn't care; I basked in the light and warmth of my newfound freedom.

We put in our orders, which took longer to fill than we had hoped. All was forgiven, though, once we were finally able to sit down to our first meal together since we had left South Dakota.

I unwrapped the quarter-pound cheeseburger and savored the feel of it between my fingers. More than a month had elapsed since I had indulged in such a meal. I know it wasn't the most nutritious food I could have ordered, but I didn't care. All I cared about was eating something piping hot and good.

I sank my teeth in the burger and began to chew. The sandwich tasted nothing like I remembered. Rather than tasting the juiciness of the meat and the sharpness of the cheese, I tasted nothing. I had the sensation of having something edible in my mouth, but my sense of taste was greatly diminished. I had to content myself with the knowledge that I was eating something other than hospital food, even if I couldn't taste it.

Mom, Dad, and I finished up at Wendy's and drove to a nearby Rainbow Foods to get groceries before going to the apartment. Dad picked out some fruits and vegetables, and I picked out some Cocoa Puffs, milk, Popsicles, and slices of Kraft American cheese. I made my selections because I knew they were among the few foods I could taste.

We finally stopped at the Cities 94 complex, collected the keys to our second-story apartment from the manager, and took the elevator upstairs. We opened the door to the warm apartment and found that it was fully furnished. It had a couch, a few chairs, and a TV in the living room, and there were a couple of twin beds in the single bedroom. There was only one wall air conditioner to serve the entire unit. The cooling would prove inadequate over the summer months, but Dad and I adjusted to the heat as best we could.

Mom helped me sort through the multiple bottles of pills and put them into my weekly pillbox. Most of the pills I had to take each day fit into the pillbox, but there were some large ones that had to remain in their bottles until I needed to take them. I also laid out my vials of saline solution on the table. I would need to keep the Hickman catheter installed for some time to come. The catheter would be flushed each day at the hospital, but I would need to flush it at home once a day.

One of the pills I received from the hospital pharmacy was morphine. I didn't expect it to have much impact on my pain, but it was better than nothing. I would learn a new meaning of pain in the following days.

Later that evening, as we all began to come down from the excitement of the day, Mom bid us adieu and returned to Brookings. I know Mom wanted to stay with us, especially during such a delicate time. But she needed to keep working to sustain us. She planned to work four ten-hour days each week and then return to the Twin Cities on Thursday evenings to join us for the weekends. And that's what she did throughout our stay.

The harsh light of day soon gave way to the softer light of evening. Dad and I were tired from all of the day's excitement, so we vegged out in front of the television. There really wasn't much on that interested either of us, other than a few programs that ushered in a new era of "reality" TV—*Survivor* and *Big Brother*. I dinked around on the computer for a few minutes and then prepared for bed. I didn't know if sleeping in the new environment would be any easier than it had been in the hospital, but at least the apartment was more like home than the hospital ever could be.

After I took the last of my meds, Dad and I retired to the bedroom. He claimed the bed closest to the window, and I took the bed closest to the door. I tried to make myself comfortable but to no avail. I was more comfortable in the apartment than I had been in the hospital, but I still couldn't sleep. I would later learn that the prednisone kept me awake.

The feeling of wanting to climb the walls and be on the move wasn't restricted to the hospital or to the daytime; such a feeling plagued me for many months to come. I realized that night that the quality of my life had risen some by getting out of the hospital—but not much.

22

Descent into Darkness

I've heard that in some things in life, such as detoxifying from various substances, the first twenty-four hours are the worst. To my dismay, that didn't seem to apply to getting out of the hospital after my bone marrow transplant. The day I left Fairview wasn't the best day I had since the bone marrow transplant, but it certainly wasn't the worst.

The following morning, I had an appointment back at the hospital. That appointment was the first of countless ones over the following three months. At least the frequency of appointments lessened over time.

Neither Dad nor I had any transportation to the hospital. Fortunately, the hospital provided a shuttle service on request. All we had to do was call, and the shuttle would pick us up patients and deliver us to the hospital. And once appointments or visits to the Phillips-Wangensteen clinic were finished, the shuttle would take us back to the apartment where we were staying. Dad called and requested the shuttle, and we took the elevator down to the main level of the apartment to wait in the early morning heat under the apartment's awning.

While we waited for the shuttle, Dad and I talked about things we'd like to see and do in the Twin Cities. We discussed was how nice it would be to have our own transportation so Dad could take me out for a drive later. Since we didn't, Dad suggested we get in touch with Uncle Gene after we returned from the clinic.

Dad and I arrived at the towering clinic about ten minutes later and caught an elevator. We entered the waiting room, and found that it was packed. To my surprise, most of the other sickly-white, bald patients were children. When I saw all the children in such a condition, my heart sank. I was sad that there were so many others like me and that many of them were children. I got a sense that the world isn't fair. It's terrible that anyone has to suffer, but it seems especially terrible when the suffering is borne by children.

With my face shielded by a surgical mask, I approached the receptionist's window and checked in. The wait to have blood drawn by one of the nurses wasn't more than a few minutes, but it seemed much longer since I was so jittery and anxious from all the medications I was on. Blood was drawn through my catheter, and the nurse weighed me before sending me back to the waiting room. I waited perhaps another twenty minutes before I was called in to see the doctor.

I had expected to see McGlave, but it was a different face I saw when the doctor walked through the door and greeted my dad and me. Rather than immediately checking my condition and evaluating my overall health, the doctor made small talk with Dad and me and seemed to make a real effort to get to know us. His pleasantries and overall calm bedside manner helped put both Dad and me at ease. And he would have the same effect on Mom in the coming weeks when she came along for visits. The doctor explained that I would see a different doctor every week. I don't fully understand why I saw the doctors on a rotating basis. It worked out all right, but there were some doctors whom I would rather not have seen.

He asked me to sit on the examining table, and he checked my skin for signs of a rash. There was something of a rash on one forearm, but the doctor assured me that it was nothing about which to be concerned.

He said that the rash was a symptom of acute graft-versus-host (GVH) disease.

Graft-versus-host disease, the doctor explained, is a condition in which the new bone marrow recognizes the host's body and treats it as though it were a foreign entity. In other words, the condition occurs when white blood cells in the new marrow attack the patient's body. The doctor said that medications such as cyclosporine and prednisone, which are immunosuppressants, are used chiefly to combat the illness. If left unchecked, GVH disease can be lethal.

The doctor said that sometimes graft-versus-host disease is beneficial for the patient. He explained that when the disease is present in a mild form, it can attack the patient's body by causing skin rashes, disrupting digestive function, and the like. While the new bone marrow attacks the patient's body, it also destroys any remaining cancer cells that may be present. So a little GVH is a good thing, he explained.

The doctor finished examining me, and then addressed the results of my blood work. He said I appeared to be progressing well, but that I required some red blood cells and platelets. So he arranged for me to have a seat in the clinic's infusion center, where Dad and I spent the next four hours as the blood products were infused into me. Before the infusion, I had asked the doctor if I could have some IV Benadryl, which he approved. It served two purposes: it would help prevent any allergic reactions I might have to the blood products. And it would sedate me and hopefully allow me to sleep, even if only for a little while. The chair in which I was sitting had a small TV attached to it, which was nice, but what I wanted more than anything else was to sleep—to be able to dream myself away from the world in which I was living. Dad sat at my side and watched TV, too, and kept me company.

It was mid-afternoon when we left the hospital. I had slept some during the blood product infusion, but I still felt pretty tired. I wanted to go home and sleep, but I suspected I couldn't because of the anxiety brought on by the steroids. Since I couldn't sleep, I suggested we get in touch with Uncle Gene to see if we could use his truck for a few days. We called Gene when we returned to the apartment, and Gene was more than happy to help. He picked up Dad and me at the apartment and took us to his house in Cottage Grove.

While we were in Cottage Grove, we visited with some cousins of mine from Waseca, Minnesota. They had come up from Waseca for the day and were eager to see how I was doing. I wish I had felt better, but I didn't really feel like visiting; I didn't have the energy. Everyone understood, though, even my younger cousins like fifteen-year-old Tom. Tom tried to talk to me about drumming. Ordinarily I would have been more than happy to banter about one of my favorite subjects, but I couldn't.

Our visit with my cousins was brief. Soon Uncle Gene offered us the keys to his red 1992 Ford pickup, and Dad and I climbed inside the truck's cab. I really didn't want to return to the apartment, so I asked Dad to drive us around the neighborhood a bit. Dad was also tired from our adventure at the clinic, but he seemed happy to comply. We cruised around downtown Minneapolis a bit and did all we could to enjoy the scenery, but I wasn't really able to enjoy myself. The heat of the day seemed to hit me especially hard, and it felt like there were always beads of sweat on my skin. I wasn't sweating profusely, but a thin veneer of sweat coated my skin. And that thin veneer always made me feel gross inside my clothes. Taking showers provided relief, but only temporarily. Anxiety from the prednisone didn't help matters, either.

We arrived back at the apartment a few minutes later and decided to peruse the mini Dairy Queen on a corner of the Cities 94 parking lot. I hadn't eaten much that day apart from the bowl of Cocoa Puffs I had before our visit to the clinic, so I ordered a hot dog with ketchup and mustard.

I worked on the hot dog on our way back up to apartment and finished it by the time we parked in front of the television. After I took my meds, I saw that Dad had tuned in to the Game Show Network. I watched TV for a while and then attempted to catch a few Zs on the couch. Unfortunately, the couch wasn't very long, so I couldn't fully lie lengthwise; I had to either prop up my head or my legs on the arms of the couch. It wasn't comfortable.

Both of us dozed for what must have been a few hours. By the time we awoke in front of the TV, it was getting toward evening. I think Dad sensed that I didn't feel well emotionally, so he asked if I wanted to walk to the Perkins up the street. I was surprised to feel that I had the strength to do so and agreed. We headed downstairs and walked to the restaurant with little trouble. We enjoyed the gentle warmth of the early evening as we walked.

We were pleased to find that the Perkins wasn't busy and that it was a clean, well-staffed facility. I still didn't have a solid sense of what I could taste, so I decided to select something simple: mozzarella cheese sticks and lemonade. The food was palatable, and the lemonade quenched my thirst nicely. After we slowly finished our meals, we could see that the sun would soon sink below the horizon, so we decided to return to the apartment. I donned my surgical mask, and we made our way back.

Once again, we turned our attention to the boob tube. Outside our open living room window, we could hear the cries and laughter of children playing in the apartment's pool. If I had been healthy, I would have loved to beat the heat by taking a dip. But I was in no condition to go swimming, so I had to experience life by the pool vicariously.

One of the first episodes of *Survivor* was on TV, and Dad watched the show from one of the living room chairs while I lay on the couch. I thought I was starting to feel drowsy and would have welcomed sleep, but suddenly I was hit with excruciating pain—pain that gripped my whole body and wouldn't let go.

I lay on the floor and writhed in agony as my limbs and trunk burned with a fire I had never felt before. The pain increased with each movement. It felt like having my entire body go into a cramp. Dad watched me for a few minutes and did what he could to help me. Neither of us really knew what to do, so I asked Dad to get me a couple of morphine pills. Dad quickly complied, and I gulped the pills and some water and tried to stifle tears as pain seared my body.

By accident, I discovered that if I lay on the floor in a certain position—flat on my back with my legs extended and my arms at my sides—the pain would lessen somewhat. In that position the pain became bearable. I still felt the pain, but I thought I could ride it out. I don't know what caused the pain or why I experienced it only once. But I'm grateful that it didn't last beyond that evening. The morphine may have lessened the pain, or it may have dissipated on its own. In the meantime, I tried to focus on the TV until I was ready to go to bed. When I sensed that it was time to head for bed, I asked Dad to help me off the floor and lead me to the bedroom. I lay face down on the bed and did the best I could to make myself comfortable, but it would be another sleepless night. I found comfort in the fact that the pain subsided as the night wore on, and I relished the thought that Mom would rejoin us in a few days.

The following morning, Dad and I prepared for what we expected would be a repeat of the previous day, except that we would drive to the clinic in Gene's truck rather than taking the shuttle—or so we planned.

Dad and I stepped out to where the truck was parked and discovered broken glass on the ground near the driver's door. Vandals had broken the driver's window and vent window. Dad and I were upset but were relieved to find that nothing had been taken from the truck. There really wasn't anything inside the truck except the CD player, and it was left intact. We reported the vandalism to the police and got in touch with Uncle Gene before we called the shuttle to take us to the hospital. The police arrived not long after, and Uncle Gene arrived later in the day. Uncle Gene was understanding about what had happened. Of course, Dad and I felt bad and suggested that Gene take the truck back to his house, and that's what we did.

After the unsettling beginning, our day progressed in much the same way as the day before. I had blood drawn, my counts were analyzed, and I received another blood and platelet transfusion after visiting with the doctor. We returned to the apartment in the late afternoon and ventured to Perkins again before retiring for the night. We were careful in heading to Perkins because both of us were concerned that the pain I experienced the night before would return. Fortunately, it never did. I had some joint pain, but it didn't seem to be connected to any kind of physical activity. To combat the pain, I took some more morphine pills.

Mom arrived late Thursday night of that week. She had been delayed for about half an hour by some road construction on Highway 212 on the western fringe of the Twin Cities. I'm sure that Mom was very tired from working and from all the driving she had done, but she appeared happy to see us, and I certainly was happy to see her.

The next day, Mom joined Dad and me as we took the shuttle to the clinic. Our visit was much the same as the previous ones, only I didn't require any blood products this time. Another doctor attended to me, and we didn't take a liking to this doctor.

When the doctor entered the room, he asked me to take my usual place on the examining table so he could look me over. Rather than begin with small talk and pleasantries, he began barking orders. He seemed to have no knowledge of the state of my treatment. He asked me about all the medications I was taking, even though the information he wanted was included in my chart.

The doctor talked for a few minutes, and then there was a break in the conversation. Mom figured it was a logical time to ask questions about how I was progressing. As Mom began speaking, the doctor cut her off. "I am talking now," he said, curtly. Mom, not one to be submissive to anyone, harshly criticized the doctor and cautioned him to not speak in such a way to her, Dad, or me. Mom's words seemed to have some effect; the doctor's overall manner didn't improve much over the following visits, but he didn't try to interrupt us again.

There was plenty of daylight left that early July day. Dad and I had run low on groceries and other supplies since Mom's last visit, so we decided it would be a good idea to do some shopping after we left the clinic. It was very warm outside, and the afternoon sun beat down on us as Dad maneuvered the family car through the mess of downtown Minneapolis traffic. There was a good deal of road construction on the city streets, and none of us was familiar with the area. But we found a store that had what we needed. In the meantime, my overall physical sense of well-being continued to worsen.

Although I hadn't eaten much the previous few days, I had a strong urge to use the restroom. I left my parents for a few minutes in the store to go to the bathroom. When I sat down on the toilet to relieve myself, I couldn't. I strained and strained but was unable to excrete the solid waste that had built up in my intestinal tract; I was severely constipated. I later learned that the constipation resulted from dehydration and from the morphine tablets I had taken. I had never had problems with my digestive tract as a result of morphine before, but taking the drug orally must have affected me differently.

I rejoined my parents, and we headed back to the apartment, where I spent the remainder of the evening dividing my time between watching TV and trying to go to the bathroom. It took perhaps two hours of straining before I was finally able to empty my lower intestine. I hadn't felt so relieved in a long time.

23

Malaise

The weeks that followed varied little. My routine was pretty well set throughout July and into early August. I visited the clinic at least once a day, had transfusions and IV antibiotics infused regularly, and saw a different doctor every week. I had bone marrow biopsies every now and then, and McGlave updated me on my progress from time to time.

To the pleasant surprise of my doctors, I recovered from the bone marrow transplant more quickly than anyone could have hoped or expected. My blood counts remained low, at least relative to what normal blood counts would be. But I was still alive, albeit weak. I experienced some GVH disease, but it was kept in check. All signs indicated that the new bone marrow was engrafting well.

In late July, when I was nearly two-thirds of the way through my tour of duty in Minneapolis, McGlave decided I was progressing well enough that I could visit the clinic every other day rather than every day. And when "every other day" fell on a weekend, McGlave permitted us to return home for a few days. I was thrilled, and so were Dad and Mom. One Friday in mid-afternoon, we packed my medicines and a change of clothes and headed back to Brookings.

We arrived in Brookings later that evening, and I only had the strength to watch some TV, take my meds (which had been reduced some from previous weeks), and head for bed. I hated the idea of going to bed at around 7:00 PM, but I didn't feel up to anything else. I was happy to be home, but I certainly didn't feel well. Still, I would rather feel ill at home than in some godforsaken hospital or apartment in Minneapolis. It was a break from my own personal hell.

Weeks before, I discovered that depression had begun to slowly creep into my life and invade my soul. The depression stemmed primarily from the physical separation from the "normalcy" of my former life. And my overall physical condition didn't help either. I had no idea of the depths of the depression at the time, but Dad and Mom were aware of it. When my parents later discussed my behavior during those dark times, both said that I seemed to go for long periods without talking; I would simply sit in silence and tolerate life as best I could. They said it was painful to see their only child, who was normally outgoing and happy, be reduced to a shadow of his former self.

My parents weren't the only ones who were aware of how I felt. Others can sometimes see us in ways that we can't see ourselves. But my condition was so dire that I, too, could sense that I was in bad shape. I felt empty. So many of the people, things, and activities about which I cared had been stripped from me. That was coupled with a lack of knowing whether my life would continue. Deep down, I still held fast to a belief that I would not die. But I felt so empty and alone that there were times I would have welcomed death. It would have ended the misery, the suffering that seemed to have no end.

I awoke that Saturday morning, completed my routine of giving myself an insulin shot and flushing my Hickman catheter, and mustered enough strength to want to do something apart from lie in bed all day. I wanted to work on my music, which I hadn't done in several weeks. Playing drums would feel good and would help me build my strength after my musculature seemed to have been destroyed.

Slowly and carefully, I made my way to the basement where my turquoise Premier XPK drums awaited me. The collection of drums and cymbals lay before me, and I climbed around my hi-hat pedal and onto the throne and did what I could to make myself comfortable. I didn't expect to be nearly as strong as I had been before I entered the hospital in September. But I wasn't prepared to have no strength whatsoever. I picked up the light pair of sticks easily enough but found that I had neither the strength nor the endurance to play a consistent eighth-note pattern on either my hi-hat or my ride cymbal. I worked on basic exercises as long as I could but was soon exhausted. And that exhaustion was disheartening. I had spent thirteen years becoming the best drummer I could be. Now, I thought I would have to rebuild my playing ability from scratch. I still retained the coordination and muscle memory required to play drums at the level I had before; I simply didn't have the strength. Feeling somewhat defeated, I stepped out from behind the drums after twenty minutes and walked back upstairs. After resting awhile, I decided to see if indulging in another passion of mine—cars—would help me feel better.

I told Mom and Dad I was going to take the NX out for a drive and then hopped in the car. I hadn't driven much in several weeks, so I knew that my coordination wouldn't be as good as when I was well. But since driving doesn't really require much strength, I didn't think I'd have a problem. I pulled the car onto the cement apron and onto the gravel driveway and then headed north on the Aurora road until it intersected with Highway 14. I cruised west to Volga and then turned around and headed back to Aurora.

I relished the sense of freedom I derived from driving alone. But the experience wasn't as pleasurable as I had expected. I still had enough strength and coordination to drive safely, but it required more effort to drive than I remembered. And it felt as though the car rode more harshly than it had before. Surely nothing with the car had actually changed since I last slipped behind its wheel. I was picking up on such sensations because of my weakened state and heightened sensitivity to my environment. I was on the road for maybe a half hour before I returned to my parents' house. I decided that that was enough driving for a while.

Sunday morning arrived before I knew it, and Dad and I returned to the Minneapolis apartment. I had another doctor's appointment the next day, and we wanted to make sure I was rested and ready. I felt fairly well—probably as well as someone who had undergone what I had could feel. Still, I didn't feel anywhere near 100 percent, but I did feel better than I had before the bone marrow transplant.

July came and went, and the furnace known as a Minnesota August set in. Doctor visits continued every other day, and each successive doctor visit with McGlave and the other doctors showed that I was making progress and was on the road to recovery. But I needed to remain in Minneapolis at least twenty more days.

There were several times in August that Dad and I, in spite of making quite a few trips to and from Brookings, developed serious cases of cabin fever. Some relief came in the form of visitors. Uncle Gene visited often, and my Uncle Frank, one of Dad's younger brothers, visited us from Devils Lake, North Dakota. Uncle Frank was always very accommodating and always quick with a grin. He helped in many ways, including driving us on one of our trips back to Brookings. There were smaller gestures as well. Once, when I was in the Phillips-Wangensteen infusion center receiving blood products, I remarked to Uncle Frank that I had lost so much weight that my pants and belt no longer fit me. Uncle Frank removed his belt and gave it to me.

Uncle Frank and Uncle Gene both helped Dad and me when our cabin fever came to a head. Dad and I both grew to hate our confinement in the apartment and our clinic visits. Dad, with Uncle Frank at his side, met with McGlave and insisted that I be allowed to go home. Dad reasoned that the remainder of my treatment could be completed in Sioux Falls. Being able to move back to South Dakota would make life easier for Dad and Mom, as well as for me. Dad and the doctor argued for a few minutes, but McGlave relented. Within a few days, McGlave had contacted doctors at Avera McKennan and arranged for the remainder of my treatment to be completed there. With Uncle Frank's and Mom's help, Dad and I moved out of our apartment. I was still short of the one hundred days required after the bone marrow transplant, but I felt all right about that. The most important thing was that I was once again in an environment in which I felt comfortable. The road to recovery lay long in front of me, but I was a lot farther along than I had been.

24

False Alarm

Dad and I arrived back in South Dakota in the middle of August, and my recovery continued uneventfully at home for the next few months. I had to visit the hospital in Sioux Falls at least once a week, and I was ordered to return to the University of Minnesota at least once a month. *No problem,* I thought to myself. *At least I'm home.*

I was now required to take shots of a drug called Neupogen to bolster my white blood cell count, which was slowly moving upward but needed some help. A few times each week, I would report to the Brookings Hospital and receive the shots. The shots seemed to work, but the injection was painful. When the drug was pushed into the muscle tissue in my upper arm, I experienced a burning, searing pain at the injection site like I had never felt before. The pain was short lived but intense.

I was still too ill to return to school, but I kept up with my buddies from school as best I could. The fall 2000 semester was a wash, but I set my sights on returning to school full-time in the spring. A little more strength returned each day. My strength seemed to gather on its own, and gradually easing back into drumming and other activities seemed to help. The road ahead remained long, but I felt like I was starting to emerge from the darkness that had enveloped me for so many months.

After leaving Minneapolis, I was only readmitted to the hospital once. Toward the end of September, I felt weak and listless and was admitted to Avera McKennan as an inpatient. I had no idea what was going on, but I had a sense that something was wrong. When I arrived at the hospital, I learned that my blood sugar had spiked. My insulin dosage was adjusted and eventually eliminated, and I received an oral medication to help control my blood sugar levels. My doctor in Sioux Falls directed me to see an endocrinologist, whom I saw a few times.

My twenty-third birthday passed quietly in November, and in early December, I began readying myself to return to the University of Minnesota for my six-month checkup. It was hard to believe that six months had passed since the transplant. I was beginning to feel more like my old self but recognized that I still had a long way to go. I also began to look more like my old self. I had put on a little weight since leaving Minneapolis, and my hair had started to grow back. My hair, which had been straight and dark, grew back curly, but was still as dark as it was the day it fell out.

The visit to Minneapolis was expected to require only a few days. Still, we packed enough clothes and supplies to last for more days if necessary. I was pleased that the visit was not supposed to last long; I had really taken a disliking to the area. And I wanted to be back in Brookings in time to greet a group of Boys and Girls Club members from the Standing Rock Indian Reservation who would visit SDSU in a few days.

I was told to expect a battery of tests when I arrived at the Phillips-Wangensteen clinic. Some of the tests, such as the lung capacity test, were easy and painless. Others were harder to endure, especially when coupled with the knowledge that something might be gravely wrong.

Apart from the lung capacity test and the usual battery of blood tests, the tests occurred after my visit with McGlave. It had been about a month since McGlave had seen me. He wanted to examine me especially thoroughly since I was at a critical point in the recovery process.

Mom and Dad remained in the waiting room while McGlave examined me. He gave me a cursory glance, his gaze fixing on my forearms, where he noticed a skin rash. The rash, which McGlave speculated was GVH, covered a greater percentage of my body than he thought it should. He stepped out of the room to allow me to undress. Not knowing what was happening or what potentially was wrong racked my insides. *Everything had gone so well up to now,* I thought. *What could be wrong?*

McGlave entered the room a few minutes later and found me sitting naked on the examination table, with my knees curled to my chest.

"Are you cold or are you just modest?" he asked nonchalantly. The truth was I was paralyzed by the prospect that something was wrong. The doctor finished his examination, excused himself so that I could get dressed, and then returned to the room with my parents. He remained calm, but I sensed that something must be wrong if he called in my parents without me requesting their presence.

Mom and Dad took chairs along one of the walls of the examining room opposite where I was seated at the examination table. Calmly, McGlave explained to us that, however unlikely, the rash could indicate that one of two things were wrong: the first was that the graft was failing in spite of all the progress it had shown over the past half year. The second was that the leukemia was returning—that I was relapsing. Our hearts sank.

McGlave assured us that everything would probably be all right but that additional tests would be required. The tests would require a longer stay in the Twin Cities. McGlave said that the key test, a biopsy of one of my salivary glands, would occur the following day. We returned to our motel, had some dinner at an adjacent diner, and retired for a night of fitful sleep. We were anxious and afraid of what the following day would reveal.

We reported to the clinic the next day. I was nervous about what would unfold, but I continued my prayers and mustered what bravery I could. I visited the bone marrow transplant clinic briefly and was referred downstairs to the dental unit. The biopsy of my salivary glands would require an incision in the inside of my lower lip so that part of one of the glands could be removed.

I waited in the busy dental area for about twenty minutes before I was escorted by a nurse to a dental chair. The dentist arrived a few minutes later, and we talked a little bit about what he was going to do. He prepared to give me some Novocain to numb the area where he was going to work. I asked if I could have some nitrous oxide to take the edge off and help calm my nerves. He said that would be no problem and sent a nurse to fetch a mask. A few minutes later, she returned and told us that no gas was available because "all the students were using it." I decided that I would need to be content with Novocain.

The doctor did what he could to calm me, and then leaned me back in the chair and asked me to open my mouth wide. He poked the inside of my lower lip with a needle, which stung briefly. The dentist waited a few minutes for the drug to take effect and then brandished his scalpel and prepared to work. He began to brush the blade of the scalpel against the inside of my mouth.

I had had many teeth filled in my life and was used to having my mouth worked on. I expected to feel pressure from the blade but not pain. Instead, I felt a sharp pain as the blade was pressed into my flesh, and I let the dentist know that I still had feeling. He injected more Novocain. A few minutes passed, and he began to press the scalpel into my lip again. I once again felt the cold steel against my flesh and tried to make him aware that I was in pain. For some reason, my message didn't get through to him, and he continued cutting. He wouldn't relent, so I raised my fist and was prepared to cuff him if necessary. He seemed to get the message. He stopped and gave me another dose of Novocain. This time, the anesthetic seemed to work, and I no longer felt pain when the scalpel was pressed against the inside of my mouth. Within a few minutes, the dentist successfully extracted part of my salivary gland, sewed up the wound, and sent me back to the bone marrow transplant clinic one more time before we headed back to Brookings.

McGlave said there was no need for us to remain in the Twin Cities any longer. He said I would receive a phone call within a few days with the results of the test.

We left the Twin Cities around three in the afternoon and returned to Brookings by eight. I drove much of the way home, grateful to feel strong enough to make such a drive. I wanted to get back to Brookings to meet with the kids from Standing Rock. I was also in a hurry to get home and be with my friends. I was almost in a state of panic and despair at that point and knew that I needed all the support I could get.

We got back to the Brookings area in time for me to meet up with Valerian, Chris, and the kids from Standing Rock. Valerian had reserved an SDSU van, and we visited on campus for a bit before we all headed to the Royal River Family Entertainment Center in Flandreau, a community about twenty-five miles southeast of Brookings. We bowled a few games there, and I did my best to bowl, be social, and have a good time. Valerian was aware of what was happening with me, but no one else really knew. It was good to be among people and to be distracted by fun activities, but I couldn't shake the sinking feeling inside. We finished bowling around ten that evening, and Valerian dropped me off at home before returning to Brookings with the rest of the group. As I stepped out of the van, one young woman asked me, "Are we ever going to see you again?" I replied, "I hope so."

I walked into the house, said good night to Mom and Dad, and retired to my bedroom. Rather than sit down at the computer and begin checking e-mail as I usually do, I fell down on my bed and began sobbing uncontrollably and unexpectedly. I don't remember ever crying so hard, but I couldn't help it. I was in a situation I had never been in before, and it was terrifying. My life hung in the balance. Intellectually, I knew that there was no point in getting upset when I didn't know for sure whether there was something about which to be upset. But I'm only human, and I was faced with the possibility of defeat—real defeat—the possibility that all I had endured, all I had suffered had been for nothing. Minutes later, Mom knocked at my door. I'm sure she wanted to comfort me, but I wanted to be left alone with my tears.

Despite the turmoil of the past few days, I slept fairly well that night. I'm sure I was exhausted from the traveling, as well as from the emotion of the trip to Minnesota and the anticipation of the news I would soon receive. I felt surprisingly well when I awoke, well enough, in fact, to go to work at the FacLab in the late morning and early afternoon. It would be good to see everyone at work, and I hoped the work would distract me from my thoughts.

I arrived at work around 10:30, and Jim and the others at ITC welcomed me back and offered words of encouragement. I didn't tell any of them about the latest round of tests; I didn't want to say anything until I knew for certain what was happening.

No faculty sought my help that day, and my solitude in the lab turned out to be a good thing. Jim was busy in another area, so I was left alone to work on video editing projects in Avid on the FacLab Macintosh. I generally felt well throughout the day but experienced mood swings like I never had before. Then again, I had never been in such a grave position. One moment, I felt as though I were about to burst into tears and descend into abject sadness. The next, my mood suddenly lifted, and I felt like laughing. A few minutes later, the pendulum swung in the other direction. I rode that roller coaster all afternoon.

Not long after I returned home that afternoon, the call came from the University of Minnesota. The person said that my test results showed there was nothing wrong with my bone marrow, and there was no sign that the leukemia was relapsing. No explanation was offered for the rash that McGlave had seen, but at the time, it wasn't important. My relief was immense, unlike anything I had ever experienced. I still didn't know whether I was out of the woods yet as far as the bone marrow was concerned, but I sensed that the trials Mom, Dad, and I had undergone in the previous few days were a major turning point.

I had no idea how much work and struggle remained ahead of me in rebuilding my life, but the tide had finally turned. I had a renewed sense that I would be all right, that I would survive.

25

Aftermath

Within a month of learning that everything was all right, I returned to school full-time. I didn't carry as heavy a credit load as I was accustomed to, but I was still back in school full-time. Along with my studies, I continued to be involved with the Native American Club. And since it was spring semester, our big project would be the powwow in mid-February.

My energy level wasn't as high as it had been before the bone marrow transplant, but that was to be expected. I remained fairly active with classes, with my job at the FacLab, and with the Native American Club. There was one time, however, that my lack of physical strength hit home.

One Saturday morning, Valerian, Chris, and I met on the third floor of Wecota Hall on campus. Valerian and the Native American Club had offices on the third floor of Wecota. The club's office needed to be moved a few doors down, and the three of us were moving things around and getting things organized. Valerian and Chris were doing much of the grunt work. Still, I wanted to do all that I could to help move larger items such as tables and chairs.

Normally, picking up chairs and sometimes even entire tables wouldn't pose a problem for me. That day I really struggled to accomplish what should have been easy, routine tasks. Both of my friends understood that I was still not healthy. They didn't expect me to do that much work. But once, my frustration at being so weak almost got the best of me.

I had tried to pick up a metal chair and move it around the room, but I didn't have the strength to do it. Chris was nearby and could see that I was struggling. He offered to take the chair from me. I kept grinning as I gingerly allowed him to take the chair from me. Inside, however, I could feel myself welling with rage. I wasn't angry with Chris or anyone else. I was angry at my physical condition, the condition to which I'd been reduced.

Do you have any idea what it feels like to be a twenty-three-year-old man, who's supposed to be the strongest he's ever going to be in his life, and he can't even pick up a chair? I wanted to scream. Instead, I screamed inside. I don't know if Valerian or Chris picked up on my frustration, but they were patient with me and did what they could to assist.

In the following months, I continued to excel in my classes. My physical abilities had been greatly diminished, but I retained most of my intellectual faculties. There were some aspects of my mind that continued to work well in spite of all I had been through, but there were others that needed a lot of healing and additional time to recover.

As the semester progressed, keeping busy helped me to keep my mind focused on the present and the future, and it helped me to keep my mind off how sick I had been and still was. At the same time, as my body grew stronger, my mental state seemed to remain a little shaky: shock and other related emotions hit me in pounding waves.

Beginning with the day I was diagnosed with leukemia, I had never really allowed myself to experience the shock, fear, and pain that one would expect to be associated with being diagnosed with a life-threatening illness. It had always been easy to remain positive about my prognosis and about the future. As I've said so before, I never seriously entertained the thought that I could die. I don't believe that such thinking was denial; I simply had an inner voice telling me that everything would be all right. As a result, I devoted my time and effort to keeping myself going, keeping myself alive, rather than dealing with the emotions. I pushed the emotions aside. All that changed when I realized I would be all right. The negative emotions and shock set in.

The spring 2001 semester ended in early May. By that time, a lot of changes had occurred in my life. I had finished another semester of college and was yet another step closer to graduating with my journalism degree. On the health front, my Hickman catheter was removed, and my medications were tapered off before June. With the tapering of the meds, my diabetes subsided, as did the anxiety associated with taking the prednisone. For the first time in months, I was medication-free.

While all appeared to be looking up, my emotional state began to nosedive. I didn't realize just how deeply I was sinking, but many bad things began to happen to me at a time when I would have thought I'd be on top of the world. I don't fully understand all that I experienced; some say it may have been post-traumatic stress disorder or withdrawal from the powerful medications I had taken. What I do understand, though, is that I'm happy that those days are behind me, and I hope I never have to go through anything like that again.

Late spring began to transition into early summer, and as temperatures rose, my spirits fell. I felt a lot of general depression during that time, but I didn't always feel bad. I experienced many nightmares, some of which were recurring, and they had common underlying themes. In each of the dreams, I would either witness other people being seriously hurt or killed, or I would be seriously hurt or killed. The dreams bombarded me in the night, and no amount of taking care of myself or seeking help dispelled them. They tormented my sleep night after night.

The nightmares continued throughout the summer and ended near the close of summer, along with many of the bad feelings I'd been having. There was no specific event or revelation that brought about the end of the dreams and the elevation of my mood. I can only attribute the gradual salving of my mind and spirit to the old adage, "Time heals all wounds."

Epilogue

As I write these words, I'm struggling to believe that so much time—nearly eight years—has passed since my initial diagnosis with leukemia. Many of the experiences seem like they occurred only yesterday; that's how close they've remained in my memory. At the same time, what I went through doesn't have the same power over me it once did. There was a time, particularly early on, when I feared I was a marked man—cancer would dog me for the rest of my life. Today, I acknowledge that there's always a chance I could relapse and fall ill again. But getting sick again isn't a big concern for me anymore. I'm more concerned now with living my life to the fullest and enjoying life to the fullest extent.

A nurse said to me, as she was preparing to infuse me with my unknown donor's bone marrow, "This will be the beginning of a new life for you." I didn't know what to make of her statement at the time, but hindsight has shown me that the nurse's words were true. My life seems now to be divided into two distinct parts: before the leukemia and after the leukemia. There are times when it's hard for me to remember what life before the leukemia was like. It's as though those days from my youth were another lifetime. Regardless, I am not the same man now that I was before and during the leukemia. And the experiences I had in going through the leukemia have, for better or worse, helped make me the man I am today.

Since those dark days, my overall health and outlook have remained positive, and there are no signs of the leukemia recurring. A few irreversible changes have occurred, including sterility from the chemotherapy and radiation and a change in my blood type from O Positive to B Positive because my donor's blood type was B Positive. But none of the changes should adversely affect the quality of my life.

My health and outlook, coupled with the love and support of my friends and family, have allowed me to accomplish much since my illness. I have earned bachelor's and master's degrees in journalism from South Dakota State University. I have published *Ethel Austin Martin: One Brave Lady*, a book the Ethel Austin Martin Program in Human Nutrition commissioned me to write. And my freelance writings and photographs have been seen by readers of newspapers, magazines, and Web sites throughout the United States and around the world. More importantly, I have traveled far on my healing journey and have continued to grow and find happiness with each passing day.

I'm not one to dwell on the past, but I acknowledge that I need to understand where I've been so that I can know where I'm going. There are many times when I question whether I learned everything I needed to as a result of going through my cancer. But the most important thing is that I'm alive and well today, and I'm doing the best I can with my life. And I hope the same will be true for all of my brothers- and sisters-in-arms who are going through what I have been through. And I pray that all of their journeys, regardless of how dark and unclear their paths, lead to better, stronger lives.

About the Author

Louis George Whitehead is a leukemia and bone marrow transplant survivor living in Brookings, South Dakota. He is the author of two published books and currently works as a freelance writer, photographer, and Web site designer. Whitehead holds bachelor's and master's degrees in journalism from South Dakota State University.

978-0-595-44522-6
0-595-44522-5